BEATING FATTY LIVER DISEASE NATURALLY

Scott A. Johnson

Beating Fatty Liver Disease Naturally / Scott A. Johnson

Cover design: Scott A. Johnson

ISBN-13: 978-1-972974-03-2

Published by Scott A. Johnson Professional Writing Services, LLC: Orem, UT

Discover more books by Scott A. Johnson at authorscott.com/shop/

DISCLAIMERS OF WARRANTY AND LIMITATION OF LIABILITY

CONTENTS

CHAPTER 1

The Silent Epidemic

What Is MASLD and Why Should You Care?

Most people find out the same way.

They go in for a routine physical—maybe it's been a few years since the last one—and their doctor orders a basic blood panel. A few days later, the results come back. Liver enzymes are slightly elevated. The doctor mentions it almost in passing: "There's a little fat on your liver. Not unusual. Let's keep an eye on it."

And that's it. No alarm bells. No clear explanation. No road map.

You go home and search online. Within ten minutes, you've encountered terms like "fatty liver disease," "NAFLD," "MASLD," "MASH," and "fibrosis." You've read that it affects hundreds of millions of people worldwide. You've also read that, in some cases, it can progress to cirrhosis or liver failure.

That's when the confusion turns to anxiety.

Here's the good news—and it's genuinely good news: You found out. And finding out early is the single most important advantage you can have. Because MASLD, especially in its early stages, is not a sentence. It's a signal. A signal that your metabolism needs attention, and that your body is ready to respond when you give it what it needs.

This chapter will give you a clear, grounded understanding of what MASLD actually is—without the fear and without the jargon. Once you understand what you're dealing with, everything else in this book will make sense.

A Name Change That Tells a Bigger Story

For nearly three decades, doctors used the term NAFLD—Non-Alcoholic Fatty Liver Disease. It was a useful label at the time, but it had a significant flaw: It defined the condition mostly by what it wasn't. "Non-alcoholic" simply meant that the liver fat wasn't caused by alcohol. It said nothing meaningful about what actually was causing it.

In 2023, a global consensus of liver specialists made a deliberate, significant shift. The new term is MASLD—Metabolic dysfunction-Associated Steatotic Liver Disease. That mouthful of a name actually matters, because every word is doing real work.

"Metabolic dysfunction" points directly at the root. This is not, at its core, a liver disease in the traditional sense. It's a manifestation of broader metabolic problems—the same ones driving type 2 diabetes, cardiovascular disease, and obesity. The liver is where we see the damage accumulate, but the trouble starts long before that.

"Steatotic" is simply the medical word for fatty. It refers to the abnormal buildup of fat (triglycerides) inside liver cells.

Why does the name change matter to you personally? Because it reframes the entire strategy. If this were purely a liver problem, you'd look for a liver treatment. But because it's a metabolic problem, the most powerful interventions address the whole system—your diet, your movement, your sleep, your hormones, your gut. That's exactly what this book is about.

What "Fatty Liver" Really Means

Every healthy liver contains a small amount of fat—that's completely normal. The problem begins when fat accumulates inside liver cells beyond a threshold of roughly five percent of the liver's total weight. At that point, the condition is called hepatic steatosis, or simply: a fatty liver.

But here's what most explanations get wrong: The fat itself isn't the primary villain. It's a symptom of a deeper problem.

Think of your liver as the body's metabolic traffic controller. It processes almost everything that comes in from your digestive system—carbohydrates, fats, proteins, alcohol, medications, environmental chemicals. It decides what gets converted to energy, what gets stored, and what gets cleared as waste. When this system is working well, traffic flows smoothly.

When metabolic dysfunction sets in—particularly insulin resistance, which we'll cover in the next chapter—the liver starts receiving more raw materials than it can efficiently process. Excess sugars and fats begin piling up inside liver cells. The liver starts doing something it's not designed to do in large quantities: It begins manufacturing fat from scratch, a process called *de novo* lipogenesis (literally, "new fat creation").

The result isn't just a liver that looks a little greasy on an ultrasound. It's a liver that's under growing stress, producing more inflammatory signals, and becoming progressively less capable of doing its many essential jobs.

Those jobs are not minor. Your liver produces bile for digestion, regulates blood sugar between meals, filters toxins from your blood, processes and regulates hormones, synthesizes proteins that govern clotting and immunity, and manages cholesterol metabolism. When it's overwhelmed, these functions begin to suffer—quietly, often invisibly, for years.

The Spectrum: MASLD, MASH, and Beyond

MASLD exists on a spectrum. Understanding this spectrum helps clarify both the urgency and the opportunity for change.

Stage 1—Simple Steatosis (MASLD): Fat has accumulated in the liver cells, but significant inflammation or scarring has not yet developed. This is by far the most common stage. At this point, the condition is highly reversible and most people have no symptoms whatsoever. Many, particularly those who make meaningful lifestyle changes, never progress beyond this stage.

Stage 2—MASH (Metabolic dysfunction-Associated Steatohepatitis): This is the more serious form, previously known as NASH (nonalcoholic steatohepatitis). "Steatohepatitis" means the liver is now both fatty and inflamed. Liver cells are being damaged. If you are at this stage, the stakes are higher—but the good news is that lifestyle intervention remains the most effective treatment available, and reversal is still absolutely achievable.

Stage 3—Fibrosis: Ongoing inflammation triggers the formation of scar tissue inside the liver. The liver can still function, but its capacity is diminishing. Earlier stages of fibrosis are still reversible with aggressive lifestyle change. Later stages become more resistant to reversal, though stabilization is possible.

Stage 4—Cirrhosis: Widespread scarring has permanently altered the liver's physical structure. Imagine a soft sponge turning into a hard, knotted rope; because the shape and texture have permanently changed, blood can no longer flow through it easily, and the liver loses its ability to function. At the advanced stage, reversal is no longer possible, though further progression can sometimes be slowed. This is why early detection and action matter so much.

Most people reading this book are in Stage 1 or early Stage 2. That's the sweet spot for intervention. The window for meaningful reversal is wide open.

A Note for People With a Normal Body Weight

Most of what you will read in this book is written with the understanding that many people with MASLD are overweight or carry excess visceral fat. That is true of the majority—but not all.

Approximately 15 to 20 percent of MASLD cases occur in people with a completely normal BMI.[1,2] This is sometimes called lean MASLD, and it is more common than most people—and many doctors—realize. If you have been diagnosed with fatty liver disease and do not consider yourself overweight, you are not reading the wrong book. You are reading a book that was written with you in mind too.

Lean MASLD tends to have a somewhat different driver profile from obesity-associated MASLD. Genetic factors—particularly variants in genes such as PNPLA3 and TM6SF2—play a larger proportional role. Fructose sensitivity, gut microbiome dysfunction, and hepatic insulin resistance (localized to the liver specifically, rather than the whole-body insulin resistance more typical of obesity) are common contributing mechanisms. Visceral fat may be present in meaningful amounts even when total body weight appears normal—this is the

"TOFI" phenomenon (Thin Outside, Fat Inside) described in Chapter 6.

The practical implications are important. If you have lean MASLD, the weight-loss-centric framing that dominates much of the public messaging around fatty liver disease does not apply to your situation in the same way. Losing body weight is not your primary goal—and aggressive caloric restriction without cause can be counterproductive. What does apply, with equal or greater force, is everything in this book about dietary quality, fructose reduction, gut health, sleep, exercise, and targeted supplementation. These interventions address the root causes of lean MASLD directly, regardless of body weight.

One additional consideration: Lean MASLD often goes undiagnosed for longer, because neither the person nor their doctor is looking for it. If you have elevated liver enzymes, a first-degree relative with liver disease, or a cluster of metabolic risk factors despite a normal weight, bring this book's lab marker recommendations in Appendix D to your next appointment and ask for a thorough metabolic evaluation.

The Scope of the Problem

MASLD is not a niche condition. It is one of the most prevalent chronic diseases on the planet.

Globally, roughly one in three to one in six adults has MASLD—an estimated 16 to 38 percent of the world's adult population.[3,4,5] In Western countries with high rates of obesity and metabolic syndrome, that number climbs higher. In the United States, conservative estimates suggest that between 80 and 100 million people are affected, with that number expected to continue to climb through 2050.[6]

What makes these numbers even more striking is how quietly the condition operates. The vast majority of people with MASLD don't know they have it. There are no pain receptors inside the liver, which means the organ can be under significant stress for years before any symptoms appear. By the time fatigue, discomfort in the upper right abdomen, or other warning signs emerge, the disease has often been progressing for a decade or more.

This is how MASLD earned the label "the silent epidemic." It spreads not through infection, but through modern lifestyle patterns—ultra-processed diets, sedentary routines, chronic sleep deprivation, and metabolic stress—conditions that define how billions of people live today.

The connection to metabolic syndrome is tight. If you have type 2 diabetes or prediabetes, obesity, high blood pressure, or dyslipidemia (abnormal cholesterol or triglycerides), your risk for MASLD is substantially elevated. MASLD, in turn, accelerates the progression of each of those conditions. These diseases don't exist in isolation—they're part of the same underlying metabolic story.

Why Most People Don't Know They Have It

The liver is famously stoic. Unlike the heart, which announces problems with chest pain, or the lungs, which signal distress with shortness of breath, the liver tends to remain silent even when it's struggling.

Early MASLD typically produces no symptoms at all. When symptoms do appear in more advanced stages, they're often vague and easy to attribute to something else—persistent fatigue, a sense of fullness or discomfort in the upper right side of the abdomen, occasional nausea, or difficulty losing weight despite effort.

Diagnosis usually happens incidentally. A routine blood test shows elevated liver enzymes—ALT and AST are the most common markers—and a doctor orders an abdominal ultrasound. The ultrasound reveals a "bright liver," indicating increased fat density. Sometimes it's discovered during imaging done for an entirely different reason.

It's worth knowing, however, that normal liver enzymes do not rule out MASLD. A significant percentage of people with fatty liver have enzymes within the normal range,[7] which is one reason the condition so often goes undetected.

If you suspect MASLD and your standard bloodwork looks normal, it's worth asking your doctor about a FibroScan (a noninvasive assessment of liver fat and stiffness), a fatty liver index calculation, or more sensitive enzyme panels. Being proactive here can make a meaningful difference.

The Metabolic Connection: Your Liver as Traffic Controller

The reason MASLD responds so powerfully to lifestyle change is that it is, at its core, a metabolic disease—and metabolism is profoundly shapable.

Here's the essential framework to keep in mind throughout this book: Your liver does not operate in isolation. It is in constant communication with your gut, your pancreas, your fat tissue, your muscles, and your brain. When any part of that system becomes dysfunctional, the liver bears a disproportionate burden.

The central driver in most cases of MASLD is insulin resistance.[8,9] When your cells stop responding efficiently to insulin—the hormone that manages blood sugar—your pancreas compensates by pumping out more of it. High circulating insulin tells the liver to ramp up fat production and reduces its ability to burn that fat for fuel. The result is that fat builds up in the liver faster than it can be cleared.

What's becoming increasingly clear, however, is that this process isn't happening uniformly throughout the day. Emerging research shows that in people with MASLD, metabolic dysfunction—especially insulin resistance—can become significantly worse at night, when the body is less able to regulate blood sugar and fat metabolism effectively.[10] This "after-hours" breakdown in metabolic control may quietly accelerate liver fat accumulation, even in people who are making progress during the day.

We'll spend considerable time on insulin resistance in the next chapter, because understanding it is the key to understanding virtually everything that follows. But for now, here's the most important concept to hold on to: MASLD is not a disease of the liver alone. It's a disease of the whole metabolic system—and the metabolic system can be restored.

The Evidence for Reversal

Let's be direct about something: MASLD, particularly in Stages 1 and 2, is one of the most responsive chronic conditions to lifestyle intervention.

The research consistently shows that losing five to ten percent of body weight—through a combination of dietary change and physical activity—leads to measurable reductions in liver fat, improved liver enzyme levels, and reduced inflammation.[11] Studies using advanced imaging have documented significant decreases in hepatic fat content within weeks of sustained lifestyle change.[12] Some participants achieve full resolution of their fatty liver.

Exercise, even without meaningful weight loss, independently reduces liver fat.[13] Dietary quality—particularly reducing fructose, refined carbohydrates, and ultra-processed foods—lowers liver fat markers significantly, often within four to eight weeks.[14] Sleep improvement reduces insulin resistance.[15] Stress management lowers cortisol, which otherwise drives abdominal and liver fat accumulation.[16]

This is not wishful thinking. It is documented, repeatable, and achievable. The chapters ahead will show you exactly how.

Start Here: Understanding Your Baseline

Before diving into the strategies that follow, it helps to understand where you're starting from. Here's a simple checklist to orient yourself.

Know Your Numbers—Key Lab Markers to Discuss with Your Doctor

- **ALT (alanine aminotransferase):** The most sensitive liver enzyme for detecting fatty liver damage. Elevated levels (above about 40 U/L in most labs) can signal liver inflammation, though normal levels don't rule out MASLD.
- **AST (aspartate aminotransferase):** Often elevated alongside ALT. The AST-to-ALT ratio can help distinguish between types of liver involvement.
- **GGT (gamma-glutamyl transferase):** A sensitive marker of liver stress, particularly from fatty liver and alcohol. Often one of the first levels to rise.

- **Fasting glucose and insulin:** Assessing insulin resistance—not just blood sugar—is critically important. Ask for a fasting insulin level; many doctors don't order it routinely.
- **Triglycerides:** High triglycerides (above 150 mg/dL) are closely linked to liver fat and insulin resistance.
- **HbA1c:** Reflects average blood sugar over three months. A value between 5.7% and 6.4% suggests prediabetes—a significant MASLD risk factor.
- **Waist circumference:** A simple, powerful proxy for visceral fat. For most adults, a waist above 35 inches (women) or 40 inches (men) is associated with elevated metabolic risk.

Three Questions to Ask Your Doctor at Your Next Visit

- "Can you check my fasting insulin level in addition to my blood glucose?"
- "Based on my labs and imaging, what stage of liver involvement do I have?"
- "What specific lifestyle changes would make the most difference for my situation?"

Key Takeaways

- MASLD (Metabolic dysfunction-Associated Steatotic Liver Disease) is the updated name for what was previously called NAFLD. The new name correctly frames this as a metabolic condition, not just a liver disease.

- Approximately 16 to 38 percent of adults worldwide have MASLD, and most don't know it. The liver rarely causes symptoms until significant damage has occurred.
- MASLD exists on a spectrum: simple steatosis → MASH (with inflammation) → fibrosis → cirrhosis. Early stages are highly reversible with lifestyle intervention.
- The liver acts as the body's metabolic traffic controller. When insulin resistance and metabolic dysfunction develop, fat accumulates in the liver as a downstream consequence.
- MASLD is fundamentally responsive to lifestyle change. Modest weight loss, improved diet quality, regular exercise, and better sleep all produce measurable improvements in liver fat and metabolic markers.
- Your most important first step: Know your numbers. Get baseline labs, understand your current stage, and use that information to guide your effort.

Now that you understand what MASLD is and why it develops, the next step is understanding the root causes—the biological and lifestyle mechanisms that drive fat into the liver in the first place. That's where the real power to reverse this condition lies.

Chapter 2 takes you there.

CHAPTER 2

Root Causes

Beyond Calories and Fat

Here's a question worth sitting with: If fatty liver were simply caused by eating too much fat, wouldn't cutting fat from your diet fix it?

For years, that was essentially the advice. Eat less fat. Cut calories. Lose weight. And while weight loss does help, millions of people who followed that guidance faithfully saw only modest improvements—or none at all. Meanwhile, people who ate plenty of healthy fats but cut sugar and refined carbohydrates showed dramatic reductions in liver fat within weeks.

Something didn't add up.

Beginning in the 1980s, dietary guidance shifted dramatically toward the idea that "fat is the enemy," driven largely by U.S. government recommendations to reduce total and saturated fat intake. These guidelines were heavily influenced by earlier research—most notably mid-20th century epidemiological studies—that linked saturated fat to heart disease, but paid far less attention to the emerging role of refined carbohydrates and sugar. In practice, this led to a widespread replacement of fats with processed, high-sugar, and high-refined-carbohydrate foods. Over time, this shift proved metabolically damaging: Instead of reducing chronic disease, it coincided with rising rates of obesity, insulin resistance, and MASLD. What was meant to protect heart health inadvertently disrupted metabolic health at a much broader level.

The problem was never just calories or fat. The problem is a complex web of metabolic dysfunction—and understanding that web is what separates a generic "eat better, move more" prescription from a strategy that actually works.

This chapter is about root causes. Not surface-level triggers, but the deeper biological mechanisms that allow fat to accumulate in the liver in the first place. Once you understand why this is happening in your body, the interventions in the chapters ahead will feel less like arbitrary rules and more like logical, targeted solutions.

The Multiple-Hit Model: Why One Cause Is Never the Whole Story

Early theories of MASLD assumed a simple linear cause: eat too much, gain fat, fat lands in the liver. This was called the "two-hit hypothesis"—first, fat accumulates; second, something triggers inflammation.[17]

We now know the reality is considerably more complex. The current understanding is what researchers call the "multiple-hit hypothesis."[18] MASLD doesn't develop from a single cause. It develops when several contributing factors converge simultaneously—genetic susceptibility, dietary patterns, hormonal dysfunction, gut microbiome imbalance, environmental exposures, and lifestyle behaviors all interacting in one system.

This is actually good news, because it means there are multiple points of intervention. You don't have to solve every problem at once.

Addressing even two or three of the core drivers can produce meaningful, measurable improvement.

Let's look at the major players.

Insulin Resistance: The Central Driver

If there is one mechanism that sits at the heart of MASLD, it is insulin resistance. Understanding it—really understanding it, not just repeating the textbook definition—changes how you think about virtually every intervention in this book.

Here's how insulin normally works. When you eat carbohydrates, your blood sugar rises. Your pancreas responds by releasing insulin, a hormone whose job is to act like a key—unlocking your muscle cells, fat cells, and liver so that glucose can enter and be used for energy or stored for later use. When everything works as designed, blood sugar rises, insulin clears it, and levels return to baseline.

Insulin resistance means those cellular locks have become sticky. The keys are still being produced—in fact, the pancreas produces more and more of them trying to compensate—but the cells aren't responding efficiently. Blood sugar stays elevated longer than it should. And the pancreas, now working overtime, keeps flooding the system with insulin.

This state of chronically elevated insulin—called hyperinsulinemia—is where the liver gets into serious trouble.

What Hyperinsulinemia Does to the Liver

High circulating insulin sends a very specific signal to the liver: Make more fat.

This process, *de novo* lipogenesis (literally "new fat creation"), is a normal metabolic function—but it's designed to operate occasionally and in modest amounts. Under hyperinsulinemic conditions, it runs in overdrive. The liver converts excess carbohydrates, particularly fructose, into triglycerides far faster than it can export or burn them. The result is progressive fat accumulation inside liver cells.

At the same time, high insulin suppresses the liver's fat-burning capacity. A healthy liver can oxidize (burn) fatty acids for fuel. Insulin blocks this process. The liver is simultaneously being told to manufacture more fat and prevented from burning the fat it already has. This is why fatty liver can develop even in people who are not significantly overweight—it's not about total calories, it's about insulin signaling.

Not All Sugars Are Equal: Why Fructose Hits the Liver Differently

Here's something most people don't realize: Two sugars with identical calorie counts can have dramatically different effects on the liver. Researchers at the Joslin Diabetes Center found that high levels of fructose in the diet inhibit the liver's ability to properly metabolize fat—and that this effect is specific to fructose.[19] Remarkably, equally high levels of glucose do not cause the same damage. In fact, glucose can actually support normal fat-burning function in the liver.

This is a critical distinction. Fructose doesn't just add fuel to the fire—it actively disables the fire department.

What makes fructose uniquely harmful is not how many calories it contains, but what it does to liver metabolism. The Joslin research showed that fructose impairs key fat-oxidation pathways, damages mitochondrial function (the liver's energy-producing machinery), and promotes fat storage. In animal studies, diets high in fructose—particularly when combined with dietary fat—produced significantly greater fatty liver changes and a measurable reduction in the liver enzymes responsible for burning fat efficiently. The liver, in essence, becomes less capable of doing one of its most important jobs.

This explains something that has puzzled researchers for years: why people who consume similar total calorie amounts but different types of sugar show such different rates of fatty liver disease.

The High-Fructose Corn Syrup Problem

Fructose in small amounts, consumed as part of whole fruit, is not a meaningful threat to liver health. Whole fruit comes packaged with fiber, water, vitamins, and polyphenols that slow absorption, support the gut microbiome, and blunt fructose's metabolic impact. The liver can handle fructose delivered this way without significant strain.

High-fructose corn syrup is an entirely different matter.

This industrially produced sweetener—derived from processed corn starch and engineered to be sweeter and cheaper than table sugar—is ubiquitous in the food supply. It shows up in sodas, energy drinks, fruit-flavored beverages, sweetened yogurts, breakfast cereals, breads, condiments, sauces, and hundreds of packaged snack products. Unlike the fructose in an apple, high-fructose corn syrup arrives in the liver concentrated, rapidly absorbed, and completely stripped of any fiber or buffering compounds that might slow its processing.

The liver has no meaningful defense against this kind of fructose flood. It arrives faster than it can be metabolized, bypasses the normal satiety signals that would otherwise limit intake, and drives *de novo* lipogenesis at a rate that whole fruit simply cannot replicate. Combine that with the damaged fat-oxidation pathways identified by the Joslin researchers, and you have a metabolic environment perfectly designed to accumulate liver fat.

Why Fructose Is Uniquely Harmful: The Missing Brake

It helps to understand why fructose is specifically more damaging to the liver than glucose because the distinction is not arbitrary and it explains why calories from different sugar sources can have dramatically different liver consequences.

When you eat glucose, the body has built-in governors. Cells down-regulate glucose uptake when they have enough energy. The pancreas monitors blood sugar in real time and adjusts insulin accordingly. There is a feedback loop that limits the rate of processing and signals fullness to the brain.

Fructose bypasses most of these governors. The key enzyme that initiates fructose metabolism—fructokinase—has no negative feedback regulation. It processes fructose at maximum speed regardless of whether the cell needs energy, regardless of whether the liver is already overwhelmed, and without triggering the satiety hormones that would normally signal fullness. As fructose is metabolized, it also depletes ATP—the cell's primary energy currency—and generates uric acid as a byproduct. Elevated uric acid independently promotes insulin resistance, increases blood pressure, and contributes to systemic inflammation.

In practical terms: When you consume a large sweetened beverage, the fructose arrives at your liver with no speed limit and no off switch. The liver cannot signal "I'm full." It simply processes as fast as it can and converts the overflow directly into fat. This is why eliminating liquid fructose—sweetened beverages above all else—produces faster, more measurable liver improvement than almost any other single dietary change. It removes the single most significant source of unregulated hepatic fuel load.

Studies have shown that just eight weeks of high-fructose feeding can induce measurable fatty liver changes even in lean individuals with no pre-existing metabolic issues.[20,21,22] This is not a slow, gradual process. The liver responds to fructose overload quickly.

Reducing or eliminating sugar-sweetened beverages—which are the single largest source of high-fructose corn syrup in the typical Western diet—is not a minor dietary tweak. It is one of the most direct and impactful interventions available for liver health. No supplement, medication, or advanced protocol comes close to the improvement achievable simply by removing liquid fructose from your daily routine.

> *Why This Matters for Your Approach. If insulin resistance is the central driver, then any strategy that lowers insulin—through diet quality, meal timing, physical activity, improved sleep, or stress reduction—directly addresses the root cause of liver fat accumulation. This is why the interventions in this book are so much more effective than simply counting calories.*

The Nighttime Problem: A Critical (and Often Overlooked) Factor

Recent research has revealed something that fundamentally reshapes how we think about MASLD—and it has important implications for when you eat, exercise, and take medications.

In a healthy metabolism, insulin secretion follows a daily rhythm. Levels are naturally higher during the day, when you're eating and active, and lower at night, when your body should shift toward fat-burning and cellular repair. This rhythm is tightly coordinated with your circadian clock.

In people with MASLD, research shows that this nighttime pattern is distinctly abnormal. Nighttime insulin secretion is lower than it should be, while insulin clearance (how quickly the body removes insulin from circulation) is unusually high.[23] The net result is a kind of metabolic vacuum during the overnight hours—a window when the liver lacks the normal hormonal signals that would otherwise support repair and fat metabolism.

Critically, this nighttime metabolic dysfunction persists even after weight loss and even after liver fat has been reduced. This tells us something important: It is not just a consequence of the disease. It appears to be a core feature of the underlying metabolic disruption.

Think of your liver like a factory. Usually, the "night shift" should be for maintenance and cleaning. In MASLD, the night shift workers (insulin) go on strike or get sent home early, but the machines keep pumping out fat anyway. This research shows that even if you "renovate" the factory (lose weight), that night shift strike still happens, making it crucial to avoid heavy meals late at night when the factory has no supervision.

What This Means for You—and Why It's Not a Reason to Lose Hope

If that last finding gave you pause, you're not alone. The idea that nighttime metabolic dysfunction persists even after weight loss and liver fat reduction can sound discouraging at first. If the problem doesn't fully resolve when things improve, does that mean your liver is permanently broken?

It doesn't. And this distinction is worth sitting with.

What the latest research reveals is that this nighttime dysfunction may be an early, underlying feature of the metabolic disruption that drives MASLD—not simply a consequence of carrying extra weight. The "night shift" problem, as it were, may have been present long before the fatty liver appeared on a scan. That makes it a root cause worth addressing directly, not a sign that the liver can't heal.

Here's what the research does not say: It does not say that people can't improve, that treatment is futile, or that the liver is beyond recovery. The same study that identified this persistence is the study pointing toward exactly the kind of targeted strategies that can work around it.

The most practical and immediately actionable of these is time-restricted eating—specifically, front-loading your calories into the earlier hours of the day and avoiding significant food intake in the hours before bed. This approach doesn't require the night shift to come back on duty. It simply stops sending deliveries when no one is there to receive them. By aligning your eating window with the hours when your metabolic machinery is most active and responsive, you reduce the fat-accumulation pressure on the liver during its most vulnerable period.

Emerging research is also investigating circadian-targeted therapies—approaches that work directly on the liver's internal clock to help resynchronize its daily rhythms.[24,25] These include specific dietary protocols, light exposure management, and pharmaceutical agents targeting circadian gene pathways. This is an active and rapidly developing area of science.

The strategies throughout this book are designed with this biology in mind. Meal timing, sleep consistency, morning-weighted activity, and stress reduction aren't arbitrary lifestyle suggestions—they're evidence-informed interventions that respect what the research now tells us about how your liver actually works across the hours of the day. You don't need a perfect metabolic clock to make meaningful, lasting progress. You need a lifestyle that works with the clock you have.

The Ultra-Processed Food Problem

Fructose doesn't arrive alone. It comes packaged in ultra-processed foods—industrially produced food products engineered for palatability, shelf stability, and low cost, but almost entirely lacking in the fiber, micronutrients, and phytochemicals that support metabolic health. These foods are not only nutritionally empty but are also deliberately designed to be hyper-palatable and easy to overconsume, making them difficult to regulate and reinforcing patterns of habitual intake.

Ultra-processed foods drive MASLD through multiple mechanisms simultaneously. They deliver refined carbohydrates and added sugars that spike insulin. They're stripped of fiber, which normally slows glucose absorption and feeds beneficial gut bacteria. They contain industrially produced seed oils high in omega-6 fatty acids, which, in excess, creates an imbalance between omega-6 and omega-3 fatty acids. Think of it like a fire department. Omega-6 provides the "alarm" to start the fire-fighting process, and omega-3 provides the "water" to put it out. Most people don't have too many alarms; they just don't have enough water. Instead of stressing about cutting out every drop of seed oil, the most effective fix for your inflammation is simply adding more omega-3s (like salmon or walnuts) to your diet and cutting back on the sugary, processed foods where those oils usually hide.[26]

Ultra-processed foods are calorie-dense but nutritionally hollow, making it easy to overconsume without feeling full. Perhaps most insidiously, they displace whole foods. Every meal built around ultra-processed products is a missed opportunity to consume the fiber, polyphenols, and healthy fats that actively protect liver cells and support metabolic function.

The practical implication is simple, even if execution isn't always easy: Reducing ultra-processed foods is one of the single most impactful dietary changes a person with MASLD can make—arguably more impactful than reducing total fat intake.

Sedentary Behavior: Sitting Is Not a Neutral Activity

Physical inactivity is not merely the absence of exercise. It is an active metabolic stressor.

Skeletal muscle is the body's largest site of glucose disposal.[27] When muscles are regularly contracted—through walking, lifting, climbing stairs, or any physical effort—they pull glucose out of the bloodstream even without insulin. This dramatically reduces the burden on your pancreas and liver. Muscle contractions also trigger the production of myokines, signaling molecules that reduce liver inflammation and improve fat metabolism directly. Think of myokines as chemical text messages that your muscles send to your liver every time they're put to work: "We're active out here—time to clean house and burn some fuel." The liver, receiving that signal, responds accordingly. When muscles are rarely contracted, those messages stop arriving, and the liver loses one of its most important external cues to stay metabolically healthy.

When you're sedentary, this entire system goes quiet. Glucose stays in circulation longer. Insulin must compensate. The liver shoulders more of the metabolic load. And over time, visceral fat—the deep abdominal fat that wraps around internal organs including the liver—accumulates.

The research on exercise and MASLD is remarkably consistent: Regular physical activity reduces liver fat independently of weight loss.[28] You don't have to lose a pound to see improvement in liver fat through exercise. This is one of the most encouraging findings in the entire field, and it's why Chapter 5 gives movement its own dedicated space.

For now, the key takeaway is this: If you sit for most of your waking hours, you are actively contributing to the metabolic environment that drives MASLD—regardless of what you eat.

Sleep Disruption and Circadian Misalignment

Sleep is not a passive state. During the overnight hours, your body carries out essential metabolic maintenance—resetting insulin sensitivity, regulating appetite hormones, clearing inflammatory debris from the brain, and orchestrating repair processes in the liver and elsewhere.[29,30,31]

When sleep is chronically short or poor in quality, metabolic function degrades in measurable, predictable ways. Just one week of insufficient sleep (five to six hours per night) has been shown to reduce insulin sensitivity by up to 25 percent in otherwise healthy adults.[32,33] Cortisol—the primary stress hormone—rises with sleep deprivation, driving up blood sugar and promoting the storage of visceral fat.

Appetite regulation also breaks down.[34,35] Ghrelin, the hormone that signals hunger, increases. Leptin, the hormone that signals satiety, decreases. The combination creates a reliable drive toward higher calorie intake, particularly of ultra-processed, high-carbohydrate foods.

Circadian misalignment—the mismatch between your biological clock and your actual daily schedule—compounds these effects. Shift workers, people who eat late at night consistently, and those with highly irregular sleep-wake patterns show markedly elevated rates of metabolic syndrome and MASLD.[36,37] The liver has its own internal clock, and it is calibrated to expect food during daylight hours and rest during darkness. Disrupting that rhythm disrupts liver metabolism directly.

Improving sleep quality and consistency is not a "nice to have" in a MASLD-reversal strategy. It is foundational. Chapter 7 provides a practical framework for addressing this.

The Gut-Liver Axis: Your Microbiome's Role

One of the most significant scientific developments in MASLD research over the past decade has been the recognition of the gut-liver axis—the dynamic, bidirectional relationship between your intestinal microbiome and your liver.

Your gut is home to trillions of microorganisms—bacteria, fungi, viruses, and other microbes—that collectively function as a metabolic organ in their own right. They help digest food, synthesize certain vitamins, regulate immune function, and produce short-chain fatty acids (acetate, propionate, and butyrate) that feed your intestinal cells. Short-chain fatty acids also act as messengers between the gut and brain, influencing the nervous system and anti-inflammatory pathways. When this ecosystem is diverse and balanced, it actively supports liver health.

When it's disrupted—a condition called dysbiosis—several things go wrong for the liver simultaneously.

First, dysbiosis is associated with increased intestinal permeability. Normally, the intestinal wall acts as a highly selective barrier, allowing nutrients to pass into circulation while keeping bacteria and their byproducts (particularly lipopolysaccharides, or LPS) contained within the gut. When this barrier becomes compromised—sometimes called "leaky gut," though that term is often oversimplified—bacterial toxins enter the portal circulation (the blood supply that goes directly to the liver). The liver, which receives this blood first, mounts an inflammatory response. Chronic low-level endotoxin exposure is now recognized as a significant driver of liver inflammation in MASLD.

Second, dysbiosis alters how the microbiome processes carbohydrates and produces short-chain fatty acids. Beneficial bacteria ferment dietary fiber to produce butyrate and other compounds that reduce intestinal permeability and liver inflammation. When fiber-fermenting bacteria are depleted—as they commonly are in people who eat low-fiber, ultra-processed diets—this protective function is lost.

Third, certain gut bacteria and fungi (like *Saccharomyces cerevisiae, Candida, Pichia kudriavzevii, Escherichia coli, Enterocloster bolteae,* and *Klebsiella pneumoniae*)[38,39,40,41,42] are particularly efficient at producing alcohol-like compounds from carbohydrates, especially sugars, through fermentation. Some individuals with MASLD harbor disproportionately high levels of these microbes, meaning their livers are dealing with a constant trickle of endogenous alcohol, even in the absence of drinking. In a very real sense, they are producing their own alcohol—without drinking a drop. That ethanol doesn't stay in the gut. It travels directly to the liver via the portal vein—the same blood supply that carries nutrients from your digestive system—where the liver attempts to process it exactly as it would alcohol consumed in a drink. The breakdown generates acetaldehyde, a highly toxic intermediate that drives oxidative stress, damages mitochondria, triggers inflammation, and activates the scarring process. Research published in 2022 by Meijnikman and colleagues measured ethanol concentrations in the portal blood of MASLD patients and concluded that gut-derived ethanol alone is sufficient to drive fatty liver development and progression.[43] People with MASLD consistently show higher levels of these ethanol-producing microbes than healthy controls, and the correlation is strongest in people who eat high-sugar, high-fructose diets—which is precisely what provides the fermentation fuel in the first place.[44] In the most pronounced cases, this process produces enough ethanol to cause measurable blood alcohol levels after a carbohydrate-rich meal, a phenomenon known as auto-brewery syndrome, and it is more common in people with MASLD than the general population. The practical implication cuts in two directions: Reducing dietary sugar starves the fermentation pathway at its source, and restoring a healthier, more diverse microbiome reduces the population of microbes doing the fermenting. Both strategies are within your reach, and together they address what is, for some people, one of the most underappreciated drivers of liver inflammation in this disease.

Restoring gut health—through dietary diversity, adequate fiber, fermented foods, and targeted probiotics—is a meaningful and underutilized strategy in MASLD. Chapter 8 is dedicated entirely to this topic.

Environmental Toxins: A Real but Often Overstated Factor

The role of environmental chemicals in MASLD deserves honest, grounded attention—neither dismissed nor sensationalized.

A class of industrial chemicals known as endocrine disruptors—including BPA (bisphenol A), phthalates, PFAS ("forever chemicals"), and certain pesticide residues—has been linked in research to metabolic dysfunction.[45,46] These compounds interfere with hormonal signaling, particularly estrogen and thyroid pathways, and some have been shown in animal and epidemiological studies to promote insulin resistance and liver fat accumulation at levels relevant to everyday human exposure.[47,48]

This does not mean that plastic water bottles are causing your fatty liver. The relationship between environmental exposures and MASLD in humans is real but modest—these are contributing factors in a multi-hit model, not primary drivers for most people.

Practical, proportionate steps—reducing plastic food and beverage containers where easy, choosing lower-pesticide produce when accessible, filtering tap water if your municipal supply has quality concerns, and avoiding heating food in plastic—reduce your total chemical burden without requiring anxiety or radical lifestyle upheaval. What this means practically is straightforward: These chemicals tend to accumulate in fatty liver tissue, where they quietly amplify the two drivers that matter most in MASLD—chronic low-grade inflammation and insulin resistance. That's not a reason for alarm, but it is a reason to take reasonable steps to reduce your exposure. Limiting endocrine-disrupting chemicals doesn't require an overhaul of your life; it simply belongs on the list of sensible, low-effort actions that collectively reduce the metabolic burden on your liver.

The goal is reasonable risk reduction, not perfection. Your diet, movement, sleep, and stress management will do far more for your liver than eliminating every possible toxin exposure.

A Practical Reduction Checklist

For those who want specific, actionable guidance beyond the general principles above, the following steps address the exposures with the most consistent evidence links to insulin resistance and metabolic dysfunction. None requires significant expense or lifestyle disruption.

Replace plastic food storage containers with glass or stainless steel alternatives. BPA and phthalates leach from plastics into food, particularly when containers are heated, scratched, or old. This is a one-time kitchen change.

Never heat food in plastic. Transfer food to glass or ceramic before microwaving. Better yet, heat your food on the stove or in the oven. Heat dramatically accelerates chemical leaching—including from containers labeled "microwave safe," which means the plastic will not melt, not that it will not leach compounds.

Filter drinking water with a carbon block filter certified to NSF Standard 58, or a reverse osmosis system. PFAS ("forever chemicals") are now detectable in the majority of municipal water systems. Standard pitcher filters do not reliably remove PFAS; NSF 58-certified systems do.

Reduce canned food consumption where practical, particularly for acidic foods such as tomatoes. Many metal cans are still lined with

BPA-containing epoxy. Fresh, frozen, or jarred alternatives are widely available.

For produce, the Environmental Working Group's annual "Dirty Dozen" list identifies the twelve items with the highest pesticide residue. Choosing organic for those specific items—while accepting conventional produce for lower-residue items—is a cost-effective strategy that does not require an all-organic commitment.

Decline printed receipts where possible, or wash hands after handling them. Thermal paper receipts are a documented BPA source via dermal absorption—a surprisingly significant exposure route for people who handle them frequently.

Personal care and household products represent a daily exposure route that most people overlook entirely. Shampoos, lotions, deodorants, body washes, and cosmetics frequently contain phthalates (typically listed as "fragrance" or "parfum," since fragrance formulas are legally protected trade secrets), parabens used as preservatives, and other compounds with documented endocrine-disrupting properties that are absorbed through skin. Household cleaning products, synthetic air fresheners, and dryer sheets add to this burden through inhalation and dermal contact. Switching to fragrance-free or "free and clear" versions of your most-used personal care products—or products that list all scent ingredients explicitly—is one of the simplest exposure reductions available. For cleaning, unscented products or basic alternatives such as castile soap, white vinegar, and baking soda replace most conventional products without sacrificing effectiveness. The Environmental Working Group's Skin Deep database (ewg.org/skindeep) allows you to search any personal care product by name and see a rated breakdown of its ingredient concerns—a useful one-time investment of fifteen minutes to audit the products you use every day.

Chronic Stress and Cortisol: The Invisible Metabolic Load

Stress is not merely a psychological state. It is a full-body physiological response with direct metabolic consequences.

When you encounter a stressor—whether physical danger, work pressure, financial anxiety, or relationship conflict—your adrenal glands release cortisol and adrenaline. These hormones mobilize energy rapidly: Blood sugar rises, heart rate increases, and stored fat and glucose are released into circulation. This is the fight-or-flight response, and in short bursts, it's adaptive and healthy.

Chronic stress, however, means chronic cortisol elevation. And sustained high cortisol does measurable damage to metabolic health: It promotes insulin resistance, drives the accumulation of visceral fat (particularly in the abdominal region and around internal organs), disrupts sleep, suppresses the immune system, and directly stimulates the liver to increase glucose production—even when blood sugar is already adequate.[49,50]

Research consistently shows that high perceived stress is independently associated with elevated liver enzymes and worse metabolic markers in people with MASLD,[51,52] even after controlling for diet and exercise. Stress doesn't just affect your behavior (leading you to eat poorly and skip workouts). It affects your biology in ways that directly promote liver fat accumulation.

This is not about eliminating stress—that's neither realistic nor necessary. It's about developing a meaningful, practiced capacity to recover from stress and increasing your resilience to stress.

Breathwork, mindfulness, time in nature, quality social connection, and adequate sleep all activate the parasympathetic nervous system, lower cortisol, and create the biological environment in which metabolic healing can occur. Chapter 7 addresses this directly.

Genetics and Epigenetics: Nature Is Not Destiny

Some people develop MASLD despite relatively modest metabolic insults. Others maintain liver health despite decades of poor habits. Genetics plays a real role—and it's worth understanding what that role actually is.

Several genetic variants have been identified that significantly increase MASLD risk.[53,54] The most well-studied is the PNPLA3 gene variant, which impairs the liver's ability to export fat efficiently. Variants in TM6SF2, MBOAT7,[55] and other genes also contribute. If you have a close family member with fatty liver disease or metabolic syndrome, there is a meaningful chance you carry some degree of genetic susceptibility.

But here's the critical nuance: Genetic susceptibility is not genetic destiny. These variants increase your risk—they don't determine your outcome. The field of epigenetics has made clear that gene expression is profoundly influenced by lifestyle. The same gene variant that accelerates fatty liver in the context of a high-fructose, sedentary, sleep-deprived lifestyle may cause minimal damage in someone who eats well, moves regularly, and sleeps adequately.

If anything, understanding your genetic susceptibility should increase your motivation, not your fatalism. People with higher genetic risk have more to gain from lifestyle optimization—and the research shows they respond just as well to intervention as those without the genetic variants.

Liver Flukes and Fatty Liver

One additional contributor worth mentioning—not because it is common in most Western populations, but because it is consistently overlooked when present: parasitic liver infections, particularly liver flukes such as *Clonorchis sinensis*, *Opisthorchis viverrini*, and *Fasciola hepatica*. These organisms cause chronic hepatic inflammation, bile duct damage, and progressive fibrosis through mechanisms entirely distinct from metabolic dysfunction—and they will not respond to dietary change, exercise, or any of the lifestyle interventions in this book. Transmission occurs primarily through consumption of raw or undercooked freshwater fish, raw watercress, or contaminated water, and risk is meaningfully elevated in people who have spent significant time in endemic regions of Southeast Asia, Eastern Europe, parts of Latin America, or sub-Saharan Africa, or who regularly eat raw freshwater fish as part of their cultural food traditions. If you fall into one of these categories and your liver enzymes remain stubbornly elevated despite genuine, sustained lifestyle effort, raising the possibility of parasitic liver infection with your doctor is a reasonable and worthwhile step. If liver flukes are suspected or identified, comprehensive evaluation is important—not just confirmation of the infection itself. Useful testing includes assessment of hepatic mitochondrial function, oxidative stress and antioxidant capacity, bile function and portal stasis markers, and a comprehensive stool analysis that includes alpha-1 antitrypsin; imaging with ultrasound is often warranted as well to assess the extent of ductal and hepatic involvement.

Reframing MASLD: A Systemic Disease, Not Just a Liver Problem

By now, a pattern should be emerging. MASLD is not a disease that originates in the liver. It is a disease that manifests in the liver as the downstream consequence of a metabolic system under sustained stress from multiple directions simultaneously.

Insulin resistance, dietary excess, inactivity, disrupted sleep, gut dysbiosis, chronic stress, environmental exposures, and genetic susceptibility don't act independently. They reinforce each other in a tangle of dysfunction. Insulin resistance worsens with poor sleep. Poor sleep promotes cravings for ultra-processed foods. Ultra-processed foods damage the gut microbiome. A disrupted microbiome drives liver inflammation. Liver inflammation worsens insulin resistance.

The loop can spin in either direction. The same interconnection that allows dysfunction to compound also means that improvements compound. Fix your sleep, and insulin sensitivity improves. Improve insulin sensitivity, and dietary changes become more effective. Improve your diet, and your gut microbiome begins to recover. A recovering microbiome reduces liver inflammation. Reduced liver inflammation improves metabolic signaling.

This is why the approach in this book is systemic rather than reductive. The goal is not to isolate one lever and pull it. The goal is to shift the whole system toward health—steadily, consistently, and in a way you can actually sustain.

Start Here: Identifying Your Root Cause Profile

Every person's MASLD has a slightly different root cause mix. The following checklist helps you identify which drivers are most significant in your own situation so you can prioritize accordingly.

Root Cause Self-Assessment

Place a check next to the factors that currently apply to you:

Dietary patterns:

- ☐ Do you consume sugar-sweetened beverages (sodas, juices, energy drinks) most days?
- ☐ Do packaged, processed, or fast foods make up a significant portion of your diet?
- ☐ Do you eat most of your calories in the evening or late at night?

Physical activity:

- ☐ Do you sit for more than eight hours per day?
- ☐ Do you engage in fewer than 150 minutes of moderate activity per week?
- ☐ Do you have a primarily sedentary job with little movement during the workday?

Sleep:

- ☐ Do you regularly get fewer than seven hours of sleep per night?
- ☐ Do you wake frequently or feel unrefreshed in the morning?
- ☐ Do you have a highly variable sleep schedule (different sleep times on weekdays vs. weekends)?

Stress:

- ☐ Do you experience chronic high stress without consistent recovery practices?
- ☐ Do you frequently feel overwhelmed, anxious, or unable to wind down?
- ☐ Does stress regularly affect your eating habits?

Gut health:

- ☐ Do you experience frequent bloating, gas, irregular bowel habits, or abdominal discomfort?
- ☐ Have you had multiple courses of antibiotics in recent years?
- ☐ Do you eat fewer than 25 grams of fiber per day?

Metabolic markers (from your labs):

- ☐ Do you have elevated triglycerides (above 150 mg/dL), low HDL, elevated fasting glucose, or a diagnosis of prediabetes or type 2 diabetes?

Environmental:

- ☐ Do you regularly eat food from plastic containers or heat food in plastic? Do you drink unfiltered tap water in an area with known contamination concerns?

The more boxes you checked, the greater the cumulative metabolic load on your liver. But here is what matters most: Each of these is addressable. Not all at once—that's not the approach—but systematically, starting with the factors that contribute most in your situation.

Prioritization Framework: Where to Focus First

If you checked items in multiple categories, use this simple hierarchy to decide where to begin. Addressing higher-priority items first creates the most leverage:

- **Priority 1—Diet quality:** Reducing sugar-sweetened beverages and ultra-processed foods produces faster, more measurable liver improvements than almost any other single change.

- **Priority 2—Physical movement:** Even a 20-minute daily walk creates meaningful metabolic benefit. Short burst of air squats—called an "exercise snack"—throughout the day are even more effective in improving metabolic function without requiring long workouts. Even a 20-minute daily walk creates meaningful metabolic benefit. Short bursts of air squats—called an "exercise snack"—throughout the day are even more effective in improving metabolic function without requiring long workouts. You don't need a perfect plan to begin: pick one, either a daily walk or three exercise snacks, and start today.
- **Priority 3—Sleep:** If you're sleeping fewer than seven hours, addressing this is non-negotiable. Inadequate sleep undermines every other intervention.
- **Priority 4—Stress management:** Establishing even one consistent stress recovery practice—breathing exercises, daily walks, mindfulness—compounds positively over weeks.
- **Priority 5—Gut health:** Increasing dietary fiber and food diversity supports gut health and requires no supplements or special protocols. Increasing the consumption of probiotics, synbiotics, and postbiotics is an important strategy as well.
- **Priority 6—Environmental reduction:** Modest, realistic steps to reduce chemical exposure without anxiety or perfection.

Key Takeaways

- MASLD is not caused by a single factor. It develops from multiple converging drivers—insulin resistance, dietary patterns, inactivity, disrupted sleep, gut dysfunction, stress, and genetics—acting on a susceptible metabolic system.

- Insulin resistance is the central mechanism. Chronically elevated insulin drives the liver to overproduce fat while simultaneously blocking its ability to burn it. Anything that improves insulin sensitivity directly addresses the root cause.
- Nighttime metabolic dysfunction is a real and underappreciated feature of MASLD. The timing of food intake and physical activity matters, not just the quantity.
- Fructose and ultra-processed foods are the most impactful dietary drivers. Reducing these produces faster liver improvement than virtually any other dietary change.
- Sedentary behavior, poor sleep, chronic stress, gut dysbiosis, and environmental toxins all contribute through distinct but interconnected mechanisms. Addressing two or three of these simultaneously produces compounding benefit.
- Genetics influences risk but does not determine outcome. Lifestyle intervention is effective regardless of genetic susceptibility—and arguably more important for those who carry risk variants.
- The most strategic first step is identifying which root causes are most active in your own situation and prioritizing interventions accordingly.

Understanding why MASLD develops is essential. But the most important question is: what does the science say about reversing it? In Chapter 3, we examine the specific biological mechanisms through which lifestyle intervention actually heals the liver—and why the research is more compelling than most people realize.

CHAPTER 3

The Science of Reversal

Why Lifestyle Modification Works—and What the Research Actually Shows

Consider two individuals. Both are diagnosed with early-stage fatty liver disease. Both have similar lab results, similar weight, similar age.

The first person leaves their appointment with a prescription and a follow-up scheduled for six months later. The second leaves with a clear, practical lifestyle plan and executes it consistently for three months.

At the six-month mark, the first person's liver fat is largely unchanged. The second person's imaging shows a forty percent reduction in liver fat. Their liver enzymes have normalized. Their insulin sensitivity has measurably improved. In some markers, their metabolic profile now resembles someone who never had fatty liver disease at all.

This is not a hypothetical. Outcomes like this are documented in the clinical literature—repeatedly, across multiple study designs, in diverse populations. And they raise a question that deserves a direct answer: If lifestyle intervention works this well, why isn't it the central focus of every conversation about fatty liver disease?

Part of the answer is that lifestyle change is genuinely harder to prescribe than a pill. It requires explanation, motivation, practical tools, and ongoing support. This book exists to provide all of those things.

But first, it helps to understand why lifestyle modification works—not just that it does, but the specific biological mechanisms through which your body begins to heal when you give it the right conditions. When you understand the mechanism, the strategy stops feeling like discipline and starts feeling like logic.

Lifestyle Modification Is Not the Alternative—It Is the Treatment

This point deserves more emphasis than it typically receives in clinical settings: Lifestyle intervention is the primary, evidence-based, guideline-recommended treatment for fatty liver disease.[56] Not a complement to medication. Not a "try this first and we'll see." The first-line therapy.

Every major hepatology society—including the American Association for the Study of Liver Diseases (AASLD) and the European Association for the Study of the Liver (EASL)—recommends sustained lifestyle modification as the foundational treatment for MASLD and MASH. This is not because pharmaceutical options don't exist or because doctors don't take the disease seriously. It's because the evidence for lifestyle intervention is, in many respects, more robust and more comprehensive than the evidence for any single drug.

No currently available medication addresses all of the root causes described in the previous chapter simultaneously. No drug improves insulin sensitivity, reduces liver fat, lowers systemic inflammation, supports gut health, improves sleep quality, and reduces visceral fat at the same time. Lifestyle intervention does all of these things—and the benefits compound with one another in ways that pharmaceutical approaches cannot replicate.

This is not an argument against medication. For some people, at certain stages of disease, medications play an important supporting role, and Chapter 11 addresses them candidly and in full. But framing lifestyle change as optional—something to attempt halfheartedly before "real" treatment begins—is both scientifically inaccurate and practically harmful. The research is clear: The most powerful lever available to most people with fatty liver disease is how they live day to day.

How Lifestyle Change Actually Heals the Liver: The Mechanisms

"Lifestyle change reduces liver fat" is a useful summary, but it glosses over the remarkable biology happening beneath the surface. Understanding the specific mechanisms—even at a basic level—changes how you think about what you're doing and why it works.

Mechanism 1: Reducing Liver Fat Directly

When you reduce refined carbohydrates, fructose, and ultra-processed foods, you remove the primary fuel source for *de novo* lipogenesis—the process by which your liver manufactures fat from excess carbohydrates. Less raw material means less fat production. The liver, no longer overwhelmed by incoming substrate, begins to export and oxidize (burn) the fat it has already stored.

This process happens faster than most people expect. Studies using MRI-based liver fat measurement have shown significant reductions in hepatic fat content in as little as four to eight weeks of dietary improvement—even without meaningful weight loss.[57] The liver is not a static storage depot. It is a dynamic, actively responsive organ, and it begins to clear excess fat relatively quickly when the conditions change.

Exercise accelerates this process through a separate but complementary pathway. Aerobic activity and resistance training both increase the liver's capacity to oxidize fatty acids by upregulating the enzymes responsible for fat burning and by improving mitochondrial function—the very function that fructose and metabolic stress had been degrading.[58] The liver's fat-burning machinery, once impaired, can be meaningfully restored.

Mechanism 2: Improving Insulin Sensitivity

Recall from Chapter 2 that hyperinsulinemia—chronically elevated insulin—is the central hormonal driver of liver fat accumulation. Reducing insulin resistance is therefore not just a desirable side effect of lifestyle change; it is one of the primary mechanisms of reversal.

Dietary improvement lowers insulin demand directly. When you eat fewer rapidly-digested carbohydrates, blood sugar rises more moderately after meals, the pancreas releases less insulin in response, and circulating insulin levels decline over time. The liver's fat-manufacturing signal quiets down.

Exercise improves insulin sensitivity through a different and powerful pathway. Skeletal muscle contractions increase the expression of GLUT4 transporters—proteins that pull glucose into muscle cells independently of insulin.[59,60] This means your muscles become better at clearing glucose from the bloodstream on their own, reducing the burden on your pancreas and liver. Regular resistance training also increases muscle mass, expanding the body's total glucose disposal capacity on a permanent basis.

Weight loss—even modest amounts—dramatically amplifies these effects. A five to ten percent reduction in body weight consistently produces measurable improvements in insulin sensitivity, liver fat, and liver enzyme levels across study populations.[61,62] For a person weighing 200 pounds, that's 10 to 20 pounds. Achievable, not extreme.

Sleep improvement and stress reduction contribute through the cortisol pathway. Lower chronic cortisol means lower fasting blood sugar, less hepatic glucose production, and reduced visceral fat accumulation—all of which ease the insulin resistance burden.

Mechanism 3: Reducing Inflammation

In simple steatosis—early fatty liver—the liver is stressed but not yet significantly inflamed. The progression to MASH (the more serious form of the disease) is driven primarily by inflammatory activation. Interrupting this inflammatory process is therefore critical not just for symptom improvement but for preventing disease progression.

Lifestyle intervention reduces liver inflammation through multiple simultaneous pathways. Omega-3-rich foods and a reduction in industrially produced seed oils shift the balance of fatty acids toward less pro-inflammatory substrates.[63] Dietary polyphenols—the compounds found in colorful vegetables, fruits, olive oil, green tea, and berries—activate anti-inflammatory signaling pathways and support the liver's antioxidant defenses.[64] Visceral fat reduction decreases the output of inflammatory cytokines from adipose tissue, which had been continuously bathing the liver in inflammatory signals.[65]

Gut microbiome restoration, which happens gradually as dietary quality improves and fiber intake increases, reduces the translocation of bacterial endotoxins (LPS) through the gut wall into portal circulation—one of the key triggers of liver inflammation described in

Chapter 2.[66] As the gut barrier heals and the population of beneficial bacteria recovers, the liver receives fewer inflammatory signals from the gut and its immune activation begins to subside.

This convergence of anti-inflammatory effects—happening simultaneously across dietary, exercise, gut, and hormonal pathways—is one of the reasons comprehensive lifestyle intervention outperforms any single targeted drug in head-to-head comparisons. No medication produces all of these effects at once.

The Goal State Has a Name: Metabolic Flexibility

Beneath every mechanism described above—reduced liver fat, improved insulin sensitivity, lower inflammation, restored gut barrier—there is a single unifying biological state that all of these changes are moving toward. It has a name: metabolic flexibility.

A metabolically flexible body can efficiently switch between burning glucose and burning fat depending on what is available and what the situation demands. After a meal, it burns glucose cleanly and stores the remainder appropriately. During fasting or exercise, it transitions smoothly into burning fat for fuel. The liver, muscles, and other tissues read these signals accurately and respond in kind.

In MASLD and insulin resistance, this flexibility is impaired. The body becomes rigidly locked into glucose-burning mode—because chronically elevated insulin keeps fat oxidation pathways suppressed, even during fasting when fat burning should naturally dominate. The liver, unable to burn its stored fat, accumulates it instead.

Every major intervention in this book restores metabolic flexibility through a different entry point. Reducing refined carbohydrates lowers chronic insulin, allowing fat oxidation to resume. Exercise activates

AMPK—the cell's master metabolic switch—which independently promotes fat burning regardless of insulin levels. Time-restricted eating creates a daily fasting window during which the transition to fat-burning can actually occur. Sleep optimization restores the nighttime metabolic repair window that MASLD disrupts.

This is why the improvements documented in lifestyle intervention studies tend to be comprehensive rather than isolated—reducing liver fat, improving insulin sensitivity, and lowering inflammation often simultaneously. They are not separate outcomes. They are multiple measures of the same underlying restoration: a metabolism regaining its ability to be flexible.

Holding this concept in mind as you read through the strategies in subsequent chapters provides a coherent frame for all of them. You are not just trying to reduce a number on a scan. You are restoring the capacity of your entire metabolic system to work the way it was designed to.

The 5 to 10 Percent Threshold: A Goal Worth Understanding

One of the most consistently replicated findings in MASLD research is the significance of a five to ten percent reduction in body weight. This threshold appears repeatedly across studies and clinical guidelines, and it's worth understanding what it actually means—and what it doesn't.

At five percent weight loss, most studies document meaningful reductions in liver fat and improvements in liver enzymes.[67] At seven to ten percent, research shows reductions in liver inflammation and early fibrosis in people with MASH. At ten percent or more, some patients achieve full histological resolution of MASH—meaning that on biopsy, the liver tissue no longer shows the characteristic signs of the disease.[68]

These are not marginal improvements. They are clinically significant outcomes that change disease trajectory.

What this threshold does not mean is that you must lose exactly five percent of your body weight before anything improves, or that weight loss is the only mechanism at work. Liver fat can decrease substantially through dietary and exercise changes even when the scale barely moves. The five to ten percent figure is a useful benchmark, not a prerequisite. People who improve their diet quality, increase physical activity, and sleep better will begin to see metabolic and liver benefits regardless of whether they've hit a specific weight target.

This distinction matters because weight loss, particularly in the early stages of lifestyle change, can be slow and nonlinear. If metabolic improvement depended entirely on reaching a weight goal, the journey would feel discouraging for many people. But because the mechanisms of reversal operate through multiple pathways simultaneously—most of which begin improving before significant weight loss occurs—the feedback from your biology tends to arrive earlier than the feedback from the scale.

> ***A Note on Realistic Expectations****. Fatty liver disease typically takes years to develop. Meaningful reversal—documented reduction in liver fat, improved insulin sensitivity, normalized enzymes—is achievable in months with consistent lifestyle change. Full resolution, where appropriate, may take longer. The goal is not perfection in ninety days; it is consistent progress over a reasonable timeline, with measurable*

> *biological markers confirming that the strategy is working.*

Why Medications Alone Are Not Enough

Several medications have demonstrated meaningful effects on liver fat, inflammation, and fibrosis in clinical trials. Chapter 11 covers the current pharmaceutical landscape in detail. But it's worth addressing directly, here, why medications alone are insufficient—not to dismiss them, but to accurately frame what they can and cannot do.

The most fundamental limitation is mechanistic. Fatty liver disease is a multi-system metabolic condition driven by insulin resistance, dietary patterns, physical inactivity, sleep disruption, gut dysbiosis, chronic stress, and in some cases environmental and genetic factors. No single drug addresses more than one or two of these drivers at a time. A GLP-1 agonist that promotes weight loss and reduces appetite does not repair the gut microbiome, improve sleep architecture, build metabolically active muscle tissue, or restore circadian insulin rhythms. It only addresses part of the problem.

There is also the question of what happens when medications are discontinued. In trials where lifestyle change accompanies medication, the benefits tend to persist and compound after the drug is stopped, because the underlying metabolic environment has genuinely improved. In trials where medication is used without lifestyle modification, benefits often diminish or reverse when treatment ends—because the root causes remain unchanged.

Long-term safety data for newer MASLD medications is still accumulating, and side effect profiles for some agents are significant. GLP-1 agonists, which have received considerable attention for their weight-loss effects, carry risks including gastroparesis (stomach paralysis), pancreatitis, gallbladder disease, potential bone density effects, and possible thyroid concerns, including thyroid tumors.[69] One of the biggest risks of rapid weight-loss drugs is that they don't just target fat—they can target your muscle, too. While the goal is to lose mostly fat, studies show that up to 40% of the weight lost on these medications can come from lean muscle.[70] Losing muscle is like shrinking your body's "engine"; it slows down your metabolism and can leave you weaker. This is why doctors emphasize that these drugs must be paired with strength training and high protein intake to ensure you're losing the "junk in the attic" and not the "frame of the house." These are not reasons to categorically avoid these medications when clinically indicated—but they are reasons not to reach for them as a first resort when lifestyle intervention is both safer and, in the long run, more comprehensive.

The most effective outcomes in MASLD management consistently come from a combination approach: lifestyle as the foundation, with medication used judiciously where the clinical picture warrants it. This book is designed to make the lifestyle foundation as strong, practical, and sustainable as possible.

The Metabolic Reset: What Is Actually Happening

The phrase "metabolic reset" gets used loosely in wellness circles, often attached to extreme detoxes or short-term protocols that promise dramatic results. The concept has real biological meaning, however—it just works differently than most of those programs suggest.

A genuine metabolic reset is not a ten-day cleanse. It is the gradual restoration of normal metabolic signaling across multiple organ systems—liver, muscle, gut, pancreas, adipose tissue, and brain—through sustained changes in the inputs those systems receive.

Here is what that process actually looks like in the body over time:

In the first two to four weeks: Liver fat begins to decline as dietary carbohydrate and fructose load decreases. Blood sugar and insulin levels start to stabilize. Energy and sleep quality often improve noticeably, even before any significant weight change.

In weeks four to twelve: Insulin sensitivity improves measurably. Liver enzymes often begin to normalize. The gut microbiome starts shifting as fiber intake increases and sugar decreases—the population of beneficial bacteria grows, and the population of harmful, ethanol-producing bacteria shrinks. Visceral fat begins to decline, reducing the inflammatory load on the liver.

In months three to six: For many people, imaging studies will show measurable reductions in liver fat at this stage. Inflammatory markers improve. If weight loss has been sustained, improvements in fibrosis markers may begin to appear. The body's hormonal and metabolic rhythms start to realign with circadian patterns as sleep and meal timing improve.

Beyond six months: The system continues to consolidate. Improvements in insulin sensitivity become more durable as muscle mass increases and visceral fat continues to decline. The gut microbiome reaches a new, healthier equilibrium. The liver, no longer under constant inflammatory pressure, has the conditions it needs for ongoing repair.

None of this happens all at once, and it doesn't happen in a straight line. There will be weeks where progress stalls, where old habits reassert themselves, where the scale doesn't move despite genuine effort. This is normal and expected. The biology does not care about perfect execution—it responds to the average of your inputs over time. Consistency, not perfection, is the variable that drives outcomes.

The Real Challenge: Adherence

The science of lifestyle intervention for fatty liver disease is genuinely encouraging. The gap between what is possible and what most people achieve is not a science problem—it is a behavior change problem.

This deserves honest acknowledgment rather than glossing over, because understanding why adherence is difficult is part of what makes it more achievable.

Most people who attempt lifestyle change for a health condition begin with high motivation and a comprehensive plan. They overhaul their diet, start an exercise program, set ambitious targets, and execute well for two to four weeks. Then something disrupts the routine—a stressful week at work, a social occasion, an injury, illness, travel—and the plan collapses. This is not a character failure. It is a predictable consequence of trying to change too many things at once in a food and lifestyle environment that is specifically designed to undermine those changes.

The behavioral science of habit formation is clear on what works. Small, specific, repeatable actions build more durable change than sweeping overhauls. Removing friction from desired behaviors—keeping vegetables pre-cut, having a consistent workout time, preparing a default healthy meal—matters more than willpower. Social support and accountability measurably improve outcomes. And self-compassion after a setback—returning to the plan without catastrophizing—is a stronger predictor of long-term success than any particular dietary or exercise strategy.

This book is designed with adherence in mind. Each chapter offers a minimal viable version of the strategy—the simplest, lowest-friction starting point that still produces meaningful benefit. The goal is to give you something you can actually do today, then build from there. Because a modest lifestyle change sustained for twelve months produces better outcomes for your liver than an aggressive program abandoned after three weeks.

Most people get this wrong: They wait until they're ready to do everything perfectly before they begin anything. The research suggests the opposite approach is more effective—start with one change, execute it consistently, allow it to become automatic, and then add the next one. The liver doesn't require a perfect plan. It requires a real one.

Start Here: Your Reversal Readiness Checklist

Before moving into the specific strategies in the chapters ahead, use this checklist to assess your starting position and set realistic expectations for your own timeline.

Readiness Assessment

- ☐ **I know my current stage:** I have had an ultrasound, FibroScan, or other imaging that gives me a baseline picture of my liver fat. (If not, this is worth requesting at your next appointment.)
- ☐ **I know my key metabolic markers:** I have recent lab results that include ALT, AST, fasting glucose, fasting insulin, triglycerides, and HbA1c. (If not, ask your doctor to add these at your next blood draw.)
- ☐ **I have identified my primary root causes:** Using the self-assessment in Chapter 2, I have a sense of which drivers—diet, inactivity, sleep, stress, gut health—are most active in my situation.

- ☐ **I have set a realistic starting goal:** Rather than committing to a complete lifestyle overhaul, I have identified the one or two changes most likely to produce early metabolic benefit in my specific situation.
- ☐ **I have a follow-up plan:** I know when I will recheck my labs—ideally at three and six months—so I can track whether the changes I'm making are producing the expected biological improvements.

What a Realistic Three-Month Timeline Looks Like

- **Month 1—Foundation:** Focus on one to two dietary changes (most commonly reducing sugar-sweetened beverages and ultra-processed foods) and establishing a consistent movement habit. Prioritize sleep if it has been consistently poor.
- **Month 2—Build:** Refine dietary quality further, increase the frequency or intensity of exercise, and add one stress reduction practice. Notice early signs of improvement: energy levels, sleep quality, morning fasting blood sugar if you monitor it.
- **Month 3—Consolidate:** Recheck key labs. By this point, most people following a consistent strategy will see measurable improvement in liver enzymes and metabolic markers. Use these results as motivation and calibration—not just a report card, but a feedback loop.

Key Takeaways

- Lifestyle intervention is the primary, guideline-recommended treatment for fatty liver disease—not an alternative to "real" treatment. It is the most comprehensive and evidence-based option available.
- Lifestyle changes work through multiple simultaneous mechanisms: reducing liver fat directly, restoring insulin sensitivity, lowering systemic inflammation, repairing the gut barrier, and rebalancing circadian metabolic rhythms.
- A five to ten percent reduction in body weight produces clinically significant improvements in liver fat and inflammation. But liver improvement—through dietary and exercise changes alone—begins before the scale moves.
- No medication addresses all of the root causes of fatty liver disease simultaneously. Medications play a supporting role in appropriate clinical contexts but do not replace the foundational impact of lifestyle change.
- A genuine metabolic reset happens gradually over weeks to months—not through short-term cleanses or extreme protocols. The biology responds to consistent inputs over time.
- Adherence is the real challenge—not the science. Small, specific, sustainable changes executed consistently outperform aggressive programs abandoned early. Start with the minimum viable version of each strategy and build from there.

The chapters ahead translate the science of reversal into concrete, practical strategies. We begin where the evidence is clearest and the impact is greatest: with food. Chapter 4 lays out a complete, evidence-based nutritional framework for liver repair—not a rigid diet, but a flexible, sustainable approach to eating that directly addresses the metabolic drivers of fatty liver disease.

CHAPTER 4

Nutrition Foundations

Eating for Liver Repair

Walk into any bookstore and count the diet books. Low fat. Low carb. High protein. Keto. Paleo. Plant-based. Carnivore. The sheer volume of competing, often contradictory advice is enough to make anyone want to eat a sleeve of crackers in defeat.

Here is the uncomfortable truth underneath all of that noise: Most popular diets work—for some people, some of the time—because most of them, in different ways, reduce processed food intake and lower the blood sugar and insulin spikes that drive metabolic disease. The specific framework matters less than most proponents claim. The underlying principles matter enormously.

There is a simpler way to state what all of that evidence points toward: Eat food that was recently alive, recently grown, or minimally transformed between the field and your plate. Not a diet identity. Not a macronutrient ratio. Not a brand. Just real, recognizable food—the kind a reasonably knowledgeable person could have made from scratch a hundred years ago. That principle, more than any specific protocol, is the axis around which this entire chapter turns.

This chapter is not about a diet. It is about a nutritional framework—a flexible, evidence-based set of principles that directly target the metabolic drivers of fatty liver disease. You will not be asked to count every calorie, eliminate entire food groups forever, or follow a rigid meal plan that ignores your preferences, culture, or schedule. You will be asked to understand what your liver needs and to make decisions that move consistently in that direction.

That distinction—between a prescriptive diet and an informed framework—is what makes this approach sustainable. And sustainability, as we established in Chapter 3, is the variable that determines long-term outcomes more than any specific dietary strategy.

Caloric Balance vs. Metabolic Quality: Getting the Framing Right

The conventional framing of diet and liver disease has long centered on caloric restriction. Eat less, create a deficit, lose weight, improve the liver. There is truth in this—weight loss does improve liver fat markers significantly, and a caloric deficit is usually required to achieve it.

But framing nutrition purely through the lens of calories misses the most actionable part of the story.

Consider two people eating the same number of calories. One gets those calories from refined grains, sweetened beverages, and ultra-processed snacks. The other gets them from vegetables, legumes, fish, olive oil, and whole grains. Their caloric intake is identical. Their liver fat outcomes, insulin sensitivity, gut microbiome composition, and inflammatory markers will be dramatically different—because metabolic quality determines how the body processes and responds to food, independent of quantity.

This is not an argument that calories don't matter. They do—particularly when the goal includes weight loss. It is an argument that metabolic quality matters more in the short term, and that improving food quality often produces spontaneous caloric reduction as a side effect, without the psychological burden of deliberate restriction. When blood sugar is stable, insulin is lower, and meals contain adequate protein, fiber, and healthy fat, appetite regulation normalizes—and people naturally eat less without counting anything.

The practical implication is this: Focus on what you eat before obsessing over how much. For most people with fatty liver disease, improving food quality will produce metabolic and liver improvements even before meaningful weight loss occurs. The quantity side of the equation tends to take care of itself as quality improves.

Macronutrient Principles: What the Evidence Shows

The three macronutrients—carbohydrates, fats, and proteins—all influence liver metabolism, but they do so differently. Understanding how each one affects the liver allows you to make more targeted choices rather than following blanket rules.

Carbohydrates: Quality and Quantity Both Matter

Carbohydrates have the most direct relationship with insulin secretion of any macronutrient, which makes them the most consequential for fatty liver disease management. But the type of carbohydrate matters as much as the amount.

Rapidly digested carbohydrates—white bread, white rice, sugary cereals, crackers, pastries, most packaged snack foods—spike blood sugar quickly and trigger a large insulin response. Consumed regularly, they sustain the hyperinsulinemic environment that drives liver fat accumulation. These are the carbohydrates most worth reducing.

Slowly digested carbohydrates—legumes, most vegetables, intact whole grains, sweet potatoes—contain fiber that slows glucose absorption, moderates insulin response, and feeds beneficial gut bacteria. These carbohydrates behave metabolically very differently from their refined counterparts, and the distinction is far more important than counting total carbohydrate grams.

The most consistently harmful carbohydrates, as established in Chapter 2, are those delivering fructose in large, concentrated doses—sugar-sweetened beverages, sweetened juices, high-fructose corn syrup in packaged foods. Reducing these produces faster, more measurable liver improvement than almost any other single dietary change.

How low should carbohydrate intake go? The research does not support a single universal answer. Significant benefit is achievable with a moderate reduction in refined carbohydrates and sugar—without going to the extremes of strict ketogenic eating, which many people cannot sustain. For those who tolerate it well and find it useful, a lower-carbohydrate approach (roughly 75 to 130 grams of carbohydrates per day from quality sources) can produce faster initial improvements in insulin sensitivity and liver fat. But this is a tool, not a requirement.

Dietary Fat: The Evidence Has Changed

For decades, dietary fat—particularly saturated fat—was cast as the primary dietary villain in metabolic disease. The picture is considerably more nuanced than that framing suggested.

Healthy fats are not harmful to the liver. Extra-virgin olive oil, fatty fish, avocados, nuts, seeds, and eggs provide fatty acids, fat-soluble vitamins, and anti-inflammatory compounds that actively support liver health. The Mediterranean diet—the most extensively studied dietary pattern for MASLD—is not low in fat. It is high in the right kinds of fat.

The fats most worth reducing in a liver-protective diet are industrially processed seed oils—corn oil, soybean oil, sunflower oil, safflower oil, and similar products that are high in omega-6 linoleic acid. These oils are abundant in ultra-processed foods and restaurant cooking. In excess, they tip the body's fatty acid balance toward pro-inflammatory substrates and have been associated with worsened liver inflammation in research models.[71,72] The debate over seed oils and their health effects continues, and to be fair, much of the research suggests a positive benefit;[73,74,75] however, processed seed oils contain high levels of a specific fat that is very unstable and highly prone to oxidation. Their unique chemical structure influences how the behave once stored in the liver—polyunsaturated fatty acids (PUFAs) contain multiple double bonds that are effectively weak points in their molecular structure. Think of saturated fats like a sturdy brick wall and seed oils like a wooden fence. In a calm environment, both are fine. However, the liver is a high-energy "hot" environment. If the liver is already stressed, the "wooden" seed oils are more likely to catch fire (oxidize) than the "brick" saturated fats. While seed oils aren't necessarily dangerous on their own, an excess of them in an already-struggling liver can provide more "fuel" for inflammation and oxidative stress.[76] If your metabolism is already stressed, these fats can "ignite," leading to chronic inflammation and damage. By swapping these for more stable fats or anti-inflammatory omega-3s, you are essentially removing the fuel that keeps the inflammatory fire burning in your liver. This does not mean small amounts are harmful, and it is not a reason to fear all cooking oil—context and dose matter. But replacing these oils with olive oil, avocado oil, or small amounts of butter where appropriate is a reasonable dietary shift.

Saturated fat from whole food sources—full-fat dairy, eggs, meat—has a more nuanced relationship with liver health than older guidelines suggested. The current evidence does not support eliminating these foods, particularly when they replace refined carbohydrates in the diet. What matters is the overall dietary pattern, not isolated nutrients in isolation.

Protein: Underappreciated and Often Under-Consumed

Adequate dietary protein is one of the most underemphasized nutritional factors in fatty liver disease management—and one of the most practically impactful.

Protein has the lowest impact on blood sugar and insulin of any macronutrient.[77,78] It is the most satiating macronutrient per calorie,[79] meaning that adequate protein intake reduces overall caloric consumption naturally. It provides the amino acids necessary for liver repair and regeneration. And it supports the preservation and growth of skeletal muscle—the tissue most responsible for insulin-independent glucose disposal.

Research suggests that higher-protein diets (1.2 to 1.6 grams per kilogram of body weight per day—0.54 to 0.73 g/lb./BW/day) support better body composition outcomes, better insulin sensitivity, and better muscle preservation during weight loss compared to lower-protein diets with the same caloric content.[80] For people losing weight to address fatty liver disease, adequate protein intake is essential to ensure that weight loss comes primarily from fat tissue rather than muscle.

High-quality protein sources include fish and seafood, poultry, eggs, legumes, Greek yogurt, cottage cheese, and lean meats. Plant-based proteins—lentils, chickpeas, tempeh, edamame—carry the additional benefit of fiber and phytonutrients. There is no compelling evidence that moderate amounts of animal protein are harmful to the liver in the context of a balanced dietary pattern.[81]

Evidence-Based Dietary Patterns for Fatty Liver Disease

Individual nutrients matter, but the most powerful dietary interventions operate at the level of overall dietary patterns—the combination and context of foods consumed together over time. Three patterns have the strongest evidence base for fatty liver disease.

The Mediterranean Diet: The Gold Standard

No dietary pattern has more consistent, more extensive evidence for metabolic benefit than the Mediterranean diet—and its effects on fatty liver disease specifically are well-documented.[82]

The Mediterranean diet is not a rigid protocol. It is a broad framework characterized by an abundance of vegetables and legumes, whole grains, fruits, nuts, seeds, and extra-virgin olive oil as the primary fat source; moderate consumption of fish, seafood, and fermented dairy; moderate wine intake (optional and not recommended as a therapeutic addition for liver health); and limited red meat and minimal ultra-processed foods.

In clinical studies, the Mediterranean diet consistently reduces liver fat, improves insulin sensitivity, lowers inflammatory markers, and produces favorable shifts in gut microbiome composition.[83] Its combination of fiber, polyphenols, omega-3 fatty acids, and monounsaturated fats addresses multiple root causes of fatty liver disease simultaneously. It is also the most extensively tested dietary pattern for cardiovascular disease,[84] type 2 diabetes,[85] and metabolic syndrome—the conditions most closely associated with MASLD.[86]

Perhaps most importantly for long-term success: The Mediterranean diet is not austere. It is built around flavorful, satisfying, culturally rich foods. The research on dietary adherence consistently shows it is one of the easier evidence-based frameworks for people to maintain over months and years. For most people with fatty liver disease, Mediterranean-style eating is the most practical dietary goal.

Lower-Carbohydrate Approaches: Fast Results, Requires Planning

Reducing carbohydrate intake—particularly refined carbohydrates and sugars—produces some of the fastest measurable improvements in liver fat of any dietary intervention. Studies comparing low-carbohydrate diets to low-fat diets in people with MASLD consistently show greater early reductions in liver fat with carbohydrate restriction,[87] driven primarily by the direct suppression of *de novo* lipogenesis.

A lower-carbohydrate approach does not require strict ketosis—a metabolic state in which the body burns fat for energy instead of glucose—to be effective. Meaningful benefit is achievable at a moderate level of carbohydrate reduction—eliminating sweetened beverages, white bread, refined grain products, and most packaged snack foods while retaining legumes, vegetables, and modest amounts of whole grains. This level of restriction is sustainable for most people and produces significant metabolic benefit.

Stricter ketogenic approaches (typically under 50 grams of carbohydrates per day) produce more rapid and dramatic reductions in liver fat and insulin levels, and they are appropriate for some individuals—particularly those with significant insulin resistance or prediabetes.[88] However, ketogenic eating requires careful planning to ensure adequate fiber, micronutrient intake, and long-term adherence. It is a powerful tool for the right person in the right context, not a universal prescription.

One practical note: The quality of fat sources matters on any lower-carbohydrate approach. A low-carbohydrate diet built around olive oil, avocados, nuts, fish, and eggs is metabolically very different from one built around processed meats and refined cooking oils. The framework is useful; the food choices within it still matter.

Intermittent Fasting and Time-Restricted Eating: Timing as a Tool

As established in Chapter 2, the timing of food intake affects liver metabolism in ways that go beyond total caloric content. This is the biological rationale for intermittent fasting and its more targeted variant, time-restricted eating (TRE).

Time-restricted eating involves condensing all food intake into a defined window—typically eight to twelve hours—and fasting for the remainder of the day. The most liver-protective version aligns this window with daylight hours: Eating begins with breakfast and ends by early evening, typically no later than 7 PM. This approach works with the liver's circadian rhythms rather than against them, ensuring that metabolic processing occurs when the liver's systems are most active and responsive.

Clinical studies on TRE in people with MASLD have shown reductions in liver fat, improvements in insulin sensitivity, reductions in body weight, and favorable changes in inflammatory markers—even when total caloric intake is not deliberately restricted.[89] Participants who confined eating to an eight-to-ten-hour daytime window showed greater metabolic improvement than those eating the same foods across a longer, less structured period.

Intermittent fasting approaches—including the 16:8 method (sixteen hours of fasting, eight hours of eating) and the 5:2 protocol (five days of normal eating, two days of significant caloric restriction)—also show benefit for liver fat and metabolic markers, though the evidence base for time-restricted eating aligned with circadian biology is more directly mechanistically supported for MASLD specifically.[90]

Intermittent fasting and TRE are optional tools, not mandatory strategies. They are particularly useful for people who tend to eat late at night, who find it easier to skip meals than to modify them, or who want to accelerate early progress. They are less appropriate for people with a history of disordered eating, those who are pregnant or breastfeeding, or those taking medications that require food for administration. When in doubt, discuss with your doctor.

Foods to Prioritize: What Your Liver Wants More Of

Rather than building a diet around restriction, it is often more effective—and more sustainable—to focus first on adding protective foods. When liver-supportive foods occupy more of the plate, the foods most worth reducing naturally occupy less of it. Notice what every food on this list has in common: Each one is either a whole food—something you could find in nature without a factory—or a minimally transformed version of one. That is not a coincidence. It is the organizing principle.

- **Fatty fish (salmon, sardines, mackerel, anchovies, trout):** Among the most impactful foods for liver health. Omega-3 fatty acids reduce liver fat, lower triglycerides, decrease liver inflammation, and improve insulin sensitivity. Two to three servings per week is a meaningful target.
- **Extra-virgin olive oil:** The primary fat source in the Mediterranean diet and one of the most studied individual foods in MASLD research. Its oleocanthal and oleuropein content provide anti-inflammatory and antioxidant effects. Use it liberally for cooking and dressings—it is not a food to use sparingly.
- **Leafy greens and cruciferous vegetables (broccoli, cauliflower, Brussels sprouts, kale, arugula):** High in fiber, folate, and sulfur-containing compounds that support liver detoxification pathways. Cruciferous vegetables in particular have been associated with reduced liver fat accumulation in research models.[91]
- **Legumes (lentils, chickpeas, black beans, edamame):** An exceptional combination of plant protein, soluble fiber, and slow-digesting carbohydrates that moderate insulin response, feed beneficial gut bacteria, and support satiety. Among the most metabolically protective foods available.
- **Berries (blueberries, strawberries, raspberries, blackberries):** Concentrated sources of polyphenols—particularly anthocyanins—with demonstrated anti-inflammatory and antioxidant effects in the liver. Their relatively low sugar content and high fiber make them the most liver-friendly fruit options.
- **Walnuts:** The nut with the strongest evidence for liver health specifically, due to their high alpha-linolenic acid (a

plant-based omega-3) content. Regular walnut consumption has been associated with improved liver enzymes and reduced liver fat in fatty liver models.[92]

- **Green tea:** Contains EGCG (epigallocatechin gallate), a potent polyphenol with documented anti-inflammatory and fat-oxidation-supporting effects in the liver. Two to three cups daily is a reasonable therapeutic target.
- **Garlic and onions:** Rich in organosulfur compounds with antioxidant and anti-inflammatory properties. Garlic specifically has been studied for its effects on liver enzymes and fat accumulation, with several trials showing modest but meaningful benefit.[93]
- **Fermented foods (plain yogurt, kefir, sauerkraut, kimchi, tempeh, miso):** Support gut microbiome diversity and the integrity of the gut-liver axis. Regular consumption has been associated with improved metabolic markers and reduced systemic inflammation.[94]
- **Eggs:** Eggs are among the most liver-supportive whole foods available—and one of the most consistently undervalued. Beyond their high-quality protein and healthy fat content, eggs are the richest common dietary source of choline, a nutrient that plays a mechanistically critical role in liver fat management. Choline is required for the liver to assemble and export fat as VLDL (very-low-density lipoprotein) particles—the vehicles through which the liver clears its fat burden into circulation.[95] One large egg provides approximately 150 mg of choline, making two eggs a meaningful daily contribution toward the 425 to 550 mg most adults require. Whole eggs are necessary for this benefit: Choline is concentrated in the yolk, not the white. Postmenopausal women have an elevated choline requirement, as estrogen normally supports the body's internal choline synthesis pathway—a pathway that declines significantly after menopause.

Foods to Minimize: What Your Liver Needs Less Of

Minimizing is not the same as eliminating. The goal here is meaningful reduction in the foods that most directly drive liver fat accumulation and metabolic dysfunction—not the creation of a permanent forbidden list that makes social eating stressful and adherence impossible.

Before getting specific, it helps to clarify what "ultra-processed" actually means—because the word is used frequently and rarely defined. The most practical working definition is this: An ultra-processed food is a manufactured product made primarily from industrially produced ingredients—refined starches, added sugars, hydrogenated fats, protein isolates, artificial flavors, artificial sweeteners, preservatives—that are assembled into something food-like but contain few or no whole food components. A useful test is the ingredient list: If it reads like a chemistry manual rather than a recipe, you are looking at an ultra-processed product. Canned tomatoes, frozen vegetables, plain yogurt, canned fish, and olive oil are processed—minimally transformed to preserve or prepare them—but they are not ultra-processed. The category below refers to the engineered products: the snack foods, sweetened beverages, flavored cereals, packaged desserts, and fast-food items specifically designed for maximum palatability at minimum cost. These products now account for more than half of calories consumed in countries like the United States. Reducing them is the single most consequential dietary shift most people with fatty liver disease can make.

- **Sugar-sweetened beverages (sodas, energy drinks, sweetened juices, flavored coffees):** The single most impactful reduction most people can make. These deliver large, concentrated doses of fructose directly to the liver with no fiber buffer, no satiety signal, and no nutritional benefit. Eliminating them—or reducing them to a rare occasional treat rather than a daily habit—produces faster liver improvement than almost any other single change.

- **Added sugars and high-fructose corn syrup in packaged foods:** Read ingredient labels. Added sugars appear under dozens of names: cane sugar, corn syrup, agave, dextrose, maltose, and many others. The goal is not zero—it is meaningful reduction, particularly in products where sugar is the dominant ingredient.
- **Refined grain products (white bread, white rice, most breakfast cereals, crackers, pastries):** These spike blood sugar and insulin with little nutritional return. Replacing them with whole grain alternatives, legumes, or vegetables where practical is one of the most metabolically meaningful swaps available. One caveat to be aware of is that brown rice has more arsenic than white rice, so in that sense white rice is a bit safer—but it comes with a tradeoff: Most white rice, especially jasmine, raises blood sugar quickly, which isn't great for fatty liver (MASLD). If you're trying to balance both concerns, the best middle ground is to not rely on rice every day, and when you do eat it, choose something like basmati rice instead of jasmine because it has a gentler effect on blood sugar. No rice is perfect, so what matters most is moderation and pairing it with protein and vegetables to keep your blood sugar steadier.
- **Ultra-processed snack foods (chips, cookies, packaged cakes, most fast food):** Calorie-dense, fiber-

poor, and engineered to override satiety signals. They displace whole foods and deliver the combination of refined carbohydrates, added sugars, and industrially produced seed oils that most directly drive metabolic dysfunction.

- **seed oils in large amounts (corn oil, soybean oil, generic vegetable oil):** Not a reason for alarm in small quantities, but worth reducing as the primary cooking fat—particularly in the context of a diet already high in processed foods, which deliver large amounts of these oils. Replace with extra-virgin olive oil or avocado oil where practical.
- **Alcohol:** Even moderate alcohol consumption is a meaningful stressor for a liver already managing fatty liver disease. The liver metabolizes alcohol with the same pathways it uses for endogenous ethanol from gut bacteria—adding exogenous alcohol compounds this burden directly. Reducing or eliminating alcohol is one of the most impactful choices a person with fatty liver disease can make. This does not require permanent abstinence for everyone, but it does warrant an honest conversation with your doctor about what level of intake is appropriate for your specific situation and disease stage.

A Sample Day of Eating: What This Looks Like in Practice

Abstract principles are useful; a concrete example is more useful. The following is a representative day of eating that aligns with the nutritional framework outlined in this chapter. This is not a prescription—it is an illustration of how the principles translate into actual meals.

Breakfast

- Two eggs scrambled in extra-virgin olive oil with a handful of spinach and sautéed mushrooms or bell peppers
- Half an avocado
- One slice of whole grain sourdough bread or a small serving of organic steel-cut oats with berries
- Green tea, hibiscus tea, or herbal tea (peppermint or ginger)

Mid-Morning (if hungry)

- A small handful of walnuts or almonds
- A serving of plain Greek yogurt with a few fresh berries

Lunch

- A large salad with mixed greens, chickpeas, cherry tomatoes, cucumber, red onion, and olive oil and lemon dressing
- A serving of canned sardines or grilled salmon alongside, or a portion of lentil soup
- Water, lemon water, or unsweetened herbal tea

Afternoon (if hungry)

- Vegetable sticks (celery, bell pepper, cucumber) with hummus
- A piece of fresh fruit—berries, an apple, or a small orange

Dinner (aim to finish by 7 PM where possible)

- Baked or pan-seared salmon or mackerel with garlic, lemon, and olive oil
- Roasted broccoli or Brussels sprouts with olive oil and a sprinkle of sea salt
- A serving of cooked lentils or a small portion of quinoa
- A glass of water with lemon

Notice what this day does: It keeps blood sugar relatively stable throughout (no large refined carbohydrate loads), delivers two servings of fatty fish, provides substantial fiber from vegetables and legumes, includes multiple polyphenol-rich foods, and uses olive oil as the primary fat. It is also, perhaps most importantly, a day built entirely from recognizable whole foods—ingredients with one-word names that exist in nature without a factory. There is no ingredient list to decode, no hidden sugar under a chemical alias, no manufactured product engineered for overconsumption. That is not an accident of the example. It is the point.

It is also flexible. The salmon can be replaced with chicken or tofu. The sourdough can be replaced with a sweet potato. The chickpeas can be replaced with black beans. The framework adapts to preferences and availability without losing its metabolic character.

The Grocery and Kitchen Reset

Environment shapes behavior more reliably than motivation does. If your kitchen is stocked with foods that undermine your metabolic health, willpower will eventually lose that battle—especially at the end of a long, stressful day. Reconfiguring your immediate food environment is one of the highest-leverage changes you can make.

The goal of a kitchen reset is not just to remove bad choices—it is to restore the kitchen to something closer to what it was before the modern food supply transformed it: a space stocked primarily with ingredients, not products. Ingredients are things you combine and cook. Products are things that arrive pre-assembled, pre-flavored, and pre-optimized to make you want more. When your kitchen contains mostly ingredients—fish, eggs, vegetables, legumes, nuts, olive oil, whole grains, spices—cooking a liver-supportive meal becomes the path of least resistance, not an act of discipline.

Remove or Reduce Friction for Poor Choices

"Friction" just means how much effort something takes. The less effort a choice requires, the more likely you are to make it—which is why the chips on the counter get eaten before the vegetables in the crisper drawer ever get chopped.

- Move sugary snacks, chips, and sweetened beverages out of easy reach or out of the home entirely
- Stop buying sugar-sweetened beverages as a household staple—replace with electrolyte water, herbal teas, or filtered water
- Clear the pantry of ultra-processed snack foods and replace with whole food alternatives: nuts, seeds, fruit, yogurt

Stock the Pantry and Fridge for Success

- Pantry: extra-virgin olive oil, canned sardines or salmon, canned chickpeas and lentils, walnuts and almonds, whole grain oats, herbal teas, canned tomatoes, garlic
- Fridge: eggs, Greek yogurt, fresh vegetables (pre-washed and pre-cut if that reduces friction), berries, avocados, lemons
- Freezer: frozen wild-caught fish, frozen vegetables (as nutritious as fresh and far more convenient), frozen berries

Simple Preparation Habits That Make Adherence Easier

- Batch-cook a pot of lentils or chickpeas at the start of the week—they become the protein and fiber base for multiple quick meals

- Pre-cut vegetables on Sunday and store them in the fridge—removing the prep friction makes it far more likely you'll eat them
- Keep a jar of mixed nuts visible on the counter—a visible healthy option is a chosen option
- Make a default weeknight dinner: a simple protein (fish, eggs, legumes), a roasted vegetable, and a drizzle of olive oil. It requires five minutes of active cooking and covers most of the nutritional bases that matter

Real-World Implementation: Making This Fit Your Life

Most people reading this chapter will not have unlimited time, a personal chef, or a food environment that makes healthy eating effortless. Here is how to apply this framework under real-world constraints.

If You Have Minimal Time

Start with the single highest-impact change: Eliminate sugar-sweetened beverages. Replace them with water, electrocyte water, or unsweetened herbal tea. This one change—which requires no cooking, no meal planning, and no new skills—begins to reduce liver fat faster than most other individual dietary interventions.

Next, add a default protein and vegetable dinner three nights per week. Canned fish and a bag of pre-washed salad greens with olive oil takes less than five minutes to assemble. A bag of frozen salmon fillets and a bag of frozen broccoli takes less than twenty minutes. Complexity is not required for metabolic benefit.

If Eating Out Is Frequent

Restaurant eating is compatible with liver-protective eating when you apply a few consistent principles: Choose grilled or baked proteins over fried; ask for olive oil and lemon instead of creamy dressings; choose vegetable sides over fries; order water or unsweetened beverages instead of sodas or juices; and skip the bread basket by default rather than by willpower.

You will not always eat perfectly in restaurants. That's expected and acceptable. The goal is a reasonable default, not flawless execution.

If Budget Is a Constraint

Eating for liver health does not require expensive specialty foods. The most impactful dietary changes—eliminating sweetened beverages, reducing ultra-processed snacks, eating more legumes and vegetables—tend to reduce grocery spending rather than increase it. Canned fish, dried lentils, eggs, frozen vegetables, oats, and olive oil are all affordable staples. Berries, when not in season, are cheaper frozen than fresh and equally nutritious.

The least expensive dietary upgrade available is replacing soda and juice with water. That single change saves money, reduces fructose load, and begins to improve liver fat markers within weeks.

> ***Most People Get This Wrong.*** *They try to change everything at once—overhaul breakfast, lunch, dinner, snacks, beverages, and supplements simultaneously in the first week. Two weeks later, exhausted and overwhelmed, they revert to their baseline and conclude that lifestyle change doesn't work for them. The evidence suggests a different approach: Pick the one or*

> *two changes with the highest metabolic leverage in your situation, execute them consistently until they're automatic, and then add the next layer. Your liver does not need a perfect diet. It needs a better one, sustained.*

✦ ✦ ✦

Key Takeaways

- The single unifying principle beneath every effective dietary strategy for fatty liver disease is the same: Eat food that is whole, recognizable, and minimally processed. All the specific guidance in this chapter—on macronutrients, dietary patterns, meal timing, and food choices—is an elaboration of that one idea.
- The most impactful single dietary change for most people is to dramatically reduce the consumption of ultra-processed food—the engineered products that make up the majority of calories in a modern diet. This does not require perfection or an expensive overhaul. It requires replacing, progressively and consistently, manufactured products with whole food alternatives. The second most impactful change: Eliminate or sharply reduce sugar-sweetened beverages.
- Metabolic quality matters more than caloric quantity in the short term. Improving food quality produces liver and metabolic benefits even before significant weight loss occurs, and tends to normalize appetite and caloric intake as a natural side effect.
- The type of carbohydrate matters more than the total amount. Rapidly digested refined carbohydrates and fructose drive liver fat accumulation; fiber-rich, slowly digested

carbohydrates from vegetables and legumes actively support metabolic health.

- Healthy fats—olive oil, fatty fish, avocados, nuts—are not harmful to the liver. They are protective. The fats most worth reducing are seed oils consumed in large amounts through ultra-processed foods.
- Adequate protein (1.2 to 1.6 g/kg/day) is underappreciated in MASLD management. It supports satiety, muscle preservation during weight loss, and insulin-independent glucose disposal.
- The Mediterranean diet has the strongest and most consistent evidence base for fatty liver disease. Lower-carbohydrate approaches produce faster early results for some people. Time-restricted eating aligned with daylight hours adds a circadian advantage that neither diet alone provides.
- Environment drives behavior. A kitchen stocked with the right foods—and cleared of the most disruptive ones—produces better outcomes than willpower alone.

✦ ✦ ✦

Nutrition is the most powerful lever in fatty liver disease management—but it is not the only one. Exercise and physical movement produce independent metabolic and liver benefits that dietary change alone cannot fully replicate. Chapter 5 explains how movement heals the liver, what types of exercise are most effective, and how to build a realistic movement habit regardless of your current fitness level.

CHAPTER 5

Movement as Medicine

Exercise That Heals the Liver

Most people assume that exercise helps fatty liver disease because it burns calories and leads to weight loss. That assumption is not wrong—but it is incomplete, and the incomplete version of the story leads to a critical misunderstanding.

The misunderstanding goes like this: If exercise helps primarily through weight loss, then exercise without weight loss is not particularly useful. And since weight loss is hard, slow, and often discouraging, some people conclude that a modest exercise habit isn't worth the effort until they're ready to commit to a more aggressive program.

The research says something quite different. Exercise reduces liver fat, improves liver enzyme levels, and lowers liver inflammation independently of weight loss.[96] You do not have to lose a single pound to begin healing your liver through movement. The biological mechanisms through which exercise helps are largely separate from those driven by caloric deficit—and they begin working from the first session.

This chapter explains those mechanisms, surveys the types of exercise with the strongest evidence for liver health, provides concrete guidance on how much is enough, and offers realistic entry points for people at every fitness level. If you do nothing else after reading this chapter, take a twenty-minute walk today. That is not a consolation prize. It is a genuine and documented therapeutic intervention.

Why Exercise Works Independent of Weight Loss

The evidence that exercise improves fatty liver disease without requiring weight loss is robust and has accumulated steadily over the past two decades. A landmark systematic review published in the *Journal of Clinical and Experimental Hepatology* analyzed multiple controlled trials and found that exercise training reduced liver fat and improved metabolic markers in people with MASLD even when body weight remained essentially unchanged.[97] This finding has been replicated across study designs and exercise modalities.

The mechanisms are specific and worth understanding because they reinforce the reasons why movement needs to be treated as a direct liver therapy rather than simply a weight management tool.

Mechanism 1: Direct Hepatic Fat Oxidation

During aerobic exercise, the liver increases its output of very low-density lipoproteins (VLDL)—the particles that export fat out of the liver into circulation for use as fuel.[98] Exercise effectively opens the liver's export channels, moving fat out more quickly than it accumulates. At the same time, the hormonal environment created by exercise—lower insulin, higher glucagon, elevated catecholamines—shifts the liver toward fat oxidation rather than fat storage.[99]

This means that every bout of aerobic exercise is directly clearing fat from the liver, regardless of whether it creates a net caloric deficit for the day.

Mechanism 2: Improved Insulin Sensitivity in Muscle

Skeletal muscle is the body's primary site of glucose disposal, and exercise is the most powerful known stimulus for improving its insulin sensitivity.[100] During muscle contractions, GLUT4 glucose transporters move to the surface of muscle cells and pull glucose in—independently of insulin. This insulin-independent glucose uptake continues for hours after exercise ends, lowering the overall demand on the pancreas and reducing the chronic hyperinsulinemia that drives liver fat accumulation.

Regular resistance training compounds this effect by increasing total muscle mass, permanently expanding the body's glucose disposal capacity.[101] More muscle means a larger metabolic sink for blood sugar—less of it reaches the liver, and the insulin burden on the entire system decreases.

Muscle Mass as a Direct Liver-Protective Factor: The Sarcopenia Connection

There is a dimension of the muscle-liver relationship that goes beyond insulin sensitivity—and it warrants explicit attention because it changes the stakes of resistance training considerably.

Low muscle mass—clinically termed sarcopenia—is independently associated with worse MASLD outcomes, higher fibrosis risk, and elevated liver-related mortality, even after controlling for body fat, BMI, and standard metabolic markers.[102] The relationship is mechanistically bidirectional, and both directions matter.

In one direction: MASLD and its associated systemic inflammation impair muscle protein synthesis by suppressing IGF-1 signaling and increasing the output of catabolic cytokines. The inflamed liver actively makes it harder to build and preserve muscle.

In the other direction: Sarcopenia worsens MASLD by reducing the body's insulin-independent glucose disposal capacity—the very mechanism that resistance training restores. Less muscle tissue means blood glucose and insulin remain elevated longer after meals, driving more liver fat accumulation. It also means lower circulating myokine levels—fewer of the beneficial signaling molecules that working muscles send to the liver to promote fat oxidation and reduce inflammation.

The clinical implication is significant: For people with MASLD, building and preserving muscle is not a cosmetic or secondary goal. It is a direct metabolic intervention with measurable liver outcomes. This is particularly important in two specific contexts. First, for people pursuing weight loss. rapid loss without resistance training and adequate protein leads to muscle loss alongside fat loss, potentially degrading the metabolic machinery being repaired. Second, for people using GLP-1 medications, research documents that 25 to 40 percent of weight lost can come from lean tissue if resistance training and protein targets are not actively maintained.[103,104] Interestingly, the most recent research suggests that about 20 percent of the lean mass loss on a GLP-1 drug may actually be from liver shrinkage as the organ sheds internal fat.

Build muscle to protect your liver. The two goals are not competing—they are the same goal.

Mechanism 3: Myokines—The Liver's Chemical Text Messages

Muscle contractions trigger the production and release of myokines—signaling molecules that travel through the bloodstream and communicate directly with the liver to reduce inflammation and improve fat metabolism.[105] Think of myokines as chemical messages that your muscles send to your liver every time they're put to work: "We're active out here—time to clean house and burn some fuel." The liver, receiving that signal, responds accordingly. When muscles are rarely contracted, those messages stop arriving, and the liver loses one of its most important external cues to stay metabolically healthy.

Irisin, IL-6, BDNF, and FGF21 are among the best-studied exercise-induced myokines with direct liver effects—reducing inflammatory signaling, promoting fat oxidation, and supporting hepatic insulin sensitivity. This myokine communication pathway is one reason why even modest exercise, well below what most fitness guidelines recommend, produces measurable liver benefits. The muscles don't need to be exhausted to send useful signals—they simply need to be regularly used.

Mechanism 4: Visceral Fat Reduction

Exercise preferentially reduces visceral fat (the deep abdominal fat stored around internal organs, including the liver) compared to subcutaneous fat (the fat directly under the skin).[106] Visceral fat is metabolically active in a harmful way: It continuously releases inflammatory cytokines and free fatty acids directly into the portal circulation that feeds the liver. As visceral fat shrinks through regular exercise, this inflammatory input to the liver diminishes.

Aerobic exercise is particularly effective at reducing visceral fat even when total body weight changes minimally. Multiple studies have documented significant visceral fat reduction with regular aerobic training in the absence of dietary change—confirming again that the benefits of exercise operate through pathways beyond simple caloric expenditure.

Types of Exercise: What Works Best for the Liver

The good news about exercise and fatty liver disease is that no single modality has a monopoly on benefit. Aerobic exercise, resistance training, and high-intensity interval training all improve liver fat and metabolic markers through partially overlapping, partially distinct mechanisms. A well-rounded program incorporates elements of at least two—but even one type, done consistently, is substantially better than none.

Aerobic Exercise: The Foundation

Aerobic exercise—sustained, rhythmic activity that elevates heart rate and breathing—has the largest evidence base for liver fat reduction.[107] Walking, cycling, swimming, jogging, rowing, and dancing all qualify. The type matters far less than the consistency and duration.

Studies on aerobic training in MASLD typically use moderate-intensity protocols: activity that elevates heart rate to roughly 50 to 70 percent of maximum (a level where conversation is possible but breathing is noticeably elevated). At this intensity, fat oxidation is maximized and the hormonal environment most favorable for liver fat clearance is created. Three to five sessions per week of 30 to 45 minutes each is the most consistently studied dose, but meaningful benefit begins at lower volumes.

Walking deserves special emphasis here, because it is the most accessible form of aerobic exercise and is often underestimated by people who associate *real* exercise with gyms and intensity. Brisk walking—at a pace that elevates heart rate and breathing without making conversation difficult—is a documented, effective intervention for liver fat reduction. A review of studies using accelerometry found that simply achieving 7,000 to 10,000 steps per day was associated with significantly lower liver fat and improved metabolic markers, independent of structured exercise sessions.

For people who are new to exercise, deconditioned, or managing joint pain, walking is not a placeholder until something better becomes possible. It is the something better. Start there.

Resistance Training: The Underutilized Prescription

Resistance training—weightlifting, bodyweight exercises, resistance bands, or any activity that works muscles against load—has historically received less attention than aerobic exercise in MASLD management. The evidence is catching up, and it is compelling.

Multiple randomized controlled trials have found that resistance training alone—without aerobic exercise and without significant dietary change—reduces liver fat, improves insulin sensitivity, lowers liver enzymes, and reduces visceral fat.[108,109] The mechanisms differ from aerobic exercise in important ways: Resistance training builds muscle mass permanently, increasing the body's long-term glucose disposal capacity. It also stimulates myokine production and improves mitochondrial function in both muscle and liver tissue.

A particular advantage of resistance training is its effect on resting metabolism. More muscle tissue means higher resting energy expenditure—the body burns more calories at rest, making weight management more sustainable over the long term. This effect compounds over months and years in a way that aerobic exercise, which does not build significant muscle mass, cannot fully replicate.

Two to three resistance training sessions per week, targeting all major muscle groups, is the evidence-based minimum. Sessions do not need to be long—thirty to forty minutes of compound movements (squats, deadlifts, rows, presses) is sufficient to produce meaningful metabolic benefit. For beginners, bodyweight exercises—squats, lunges, push-ups, and planks—provide an effective entry point with no equipment required.

High-Intensity Interval Training: Efficient but Demanding

High-intensity interval training (HIIT) involves alternating short bursts of high-effort activity with recovery periods. A typical protocol might be twenty to thirty seconds of near-maximal effort followed by sixty to ninety seconds of easy movement, repeated for fifteen to twenty minutes total.

HIIT produces comparable or superior improvements in liver fat and insulin sensitivity to moderate-intensity continuous exercise in less total time.[110] For people with busy schedules, this time efficiency is a genuine practical advantage. HIIT also produces a pronounced post-exercise metabolic effect—elevated fat oxidation and oxygen consumption that continues for hours after the session ends.[111]

The limitation of HIIT is its physical demand. It requires a baseline level of fitness, places significant stress on joints and the cardiovascular system, and carries higher injury risk than lower-intensity modalities. It is not an appropriate starting point for people who are significantly deconditioned or managing cardiovascular disease or joint issues. For those who are ready for it, two HIIT sessions per week—interspersed with lower-intensity activity on other days—is an effective, time-efficient protocol.

The Air Squat: A Surprisingly Powerful Micro-Intervention

Recent research has highlighted the metabolic value of brief, structured movement breaks throughout the day—and the bodyweight squat turns out to be one of the most efficient tools available for this purpose.

A study published in *Scientific Reports* found that short bouts of air squats performed at regular intervals throughout the day efficiently improved cardiovascular fitness, muscle strength, and metabolic function—without requiring long workouts or special equipment.[112] The squat engages the largest muscle groups in the body (quadriceps, hamstrings, glutes), generates a strong myokine response, and drives meaningful glucose uptake in muscle tissue—all within a movement that requires no gym, no equipment, and can be performed in thirty seconds at a desk.

The practical application: three sets of ten to fifteen air squats, performed two to three times throughout the workday, delivers a cumulative metabolic signal that interrupts the harmful effects of prolonged sitting. This is not a replacement for structured exercise—it is a complement to it, and a particularly valuable one for people who work desk jobs and struggle to find time for formal workouts. A few dozen squats distributed through the day will not transform your fitness, but they will meaningfully alter your metabolic environment in ways that benefit the liver.

Dose-Response: How Much Is Actually Enough?

This is the question most people want answered, and the honest answer is more encouraging than most people expect.

Current guidelines for MASLD management recommend 150 to 300 minutes of moderate-intensity aerobic activity per week, combined with two to three resistance training sessions. This is the dose at which the most robust liver benefits have been documented in clinical trials. But that recommendation describes an optimal target, not a minimum threshold.

The dose-response relationship between exercise and liver health is not binary. It is a curve—and even small amounts of movement, well below the guideline recommendation, produce measurable benefit compared to sedentary behavior. Studies have documented significant improvements in liver fat and insulin sensitivity with as little as 75 minutes of moderate activity per week. The incremental benefit continues to accumulate as volume increases, but the steepest part of the improvement curve occurs in the transition from sedentary to lightly active.

In practical terms: Going from zero structured exercise to three twenty-minute walks per week produces more liver benefit than going from three workouts per week to five. The largest gains are available to those who are currently sedentary—which means the barrier to entry is lower than it appears.

> ***The Most Important Exercise Principle in This Book.*** *Something is always better than nothing. Perfect is the enemy of good. A twenty-minute walk done consistently five days a week will produce better liver outcomes over twelve months than an ambitious training program that gets abandoned after three weeks. Design your exercise habit around what you will*

> *actually do, not around what you think you should theoretically be doing.*

NEAT: The Hidden Metabolic Variable

NEAT stands for non-exercise activity thermogenesis—the energy your body expends on all physical movement that is not deliberate exercise. Walking to the mailbox, climbing stairs, fidgeting, standing while on a phone call, doing household tasks, walking through a parking lot rather than circling for the closest spot. Individually trivial. Collectively enormous.

Research has established that NEAT accounts for the majority of the physical activity energy expenditure differences between individuals. Two people can have identical formal exercise habits and differ by 500 to 1,000 calories per day in total energy expenditure—simply because one person moves considerably more throughout their non-exercise hours. This difference, compounded over months and years, has profound effects on body composition, insulin sensitivity, and liver fat.

The practical implication of NEAT is that your movement habits outside the gym matter as much as—or more than—your formal exercise sessions. And they are far more easily managed. You cannot easily add an extra hour of exercise to a packed schedule. You can park farther away, take the stairs, walk while taking phone calls, stand at your desk for part of the workday, and get up from your chair every hour for a brief walk. These micro-movements add up to a metabolic environment that is meaningfully different from a fully sedentary one.

One particularly useful NEAT target is interrupting prolonged sitting. Research shows that sitting continuously for more than sixty to ninety minutes begins to impair glucose metabolism and insulin sensitivity in ways that a single daily exercise session cannot fully counteract.[113] Standing up and moving for two to five minutes every hour—even just walking to get a glass of water—measurably reduces these negative effects. Set a timer if necessary. The interruption matters.

The Post-Meal Window: The Highest-Leverage Timing for Brief Movement

Among all timing strategies for physical activity, one stands out for its disproportionate metabolic impact relative to the effort required: walking for 10 to 15 minutes immediately after a meal.

Research consistently shows that brief post-meal walks reduce postprandial blood glucose by 10 to 30 percent and lower the corresponding insulin response.[114,115,116] Even more impressive, one minute of stair climbing and descending after a meal improves both glucose and insulin responses within one to three minutes.[117] The mechanism requires no special fitness level and no equipment. When muscles contract during walking or stair climbing and descending, they pull glucose from the bloodstream directly and independently of insulin—through GLUT4 transporter activation in muscle cells. Immediately after eating, blood glucose is rising and the liver is beginning to process the meal's substrate load. A short walk at this moment intercepts a portion of that glucose before it triggers a large insulin spike, reducing the very hyperinsulinemic environment that drives liver fat accumulation.

Three 10-minute walks per day—one after each main meal—deliver a cumulative metabolic effect that some research suggests exceeds that of a single 30-minute walk taken at a neutral time during the day. For people managing insulin resistance and MASLD, the timing matters alongside the movement itself.

This is one of the most accessible interventions in this entire book. It requires no gym, no special clothing, no baseline fitness level, and no additional time beyond what meals naturally create. A short loop around the block, a circuit through the building, or deliberate movement within the home is sufficient. If you implement one new walking habit from this chapter, starting with the post-dinner walk is usually the most practical—since the evening meal is typically the largest, and its postprandial glucose peak the most metabolically significant.

Personalized Plans: From Beginner to Advanced

The following plans are designed as starting frameworks, not rigid prescriptions. Adjust them to your current fitness level, health status, schedule, and preferences. The goal is a sustainable habit you will actually maintain—not the most impressive program on paper.

Beginner Plan—"Start Where You Are"

Appropriate for: People currently sedentary or largely inactive, those managing joint pain or cardiovascular concerns, anyone returning to activity after a significant break.

- **Week 1 to 2:** Two to three 15-minute brisk walks per day. No gym required. Focus on consistency over intensity.
- **Week 3 to 4:** Extend walks to 20 to 25 minutes. Add two sessions of ten bodyweight squats, ten chair-assisted lunges, and ten wall push-ups. These can be done at home in under ten minutes.
- **Week 5 to 8:** Work toward 30-minute walks five days per week. Add a third resistance session. Introduce movement breaks every hour at work: a brief walk or two to three sets of air squats.

By the end of eight weeks, a beginner following this plan will have established a consistent movement habit, begun building foundational strength, and already generated measurable myokine-driven liver benefits—without a gym membership or a single piece of equipment.

Intermediate Plan—"Build and Consolidate"

Appropriate for: People who already walk regularly or exercise occasionally but have not established a consistent structured program.

- **Aerobic:** Four sessions per week of 30 to 40 minutes of moderate-intensity aerobic activity—brisk walking, cycling, swimming, or any preferred modality. Heart rate elevated to the point where conversation is possible but breathing is noticeably elevated.
- **Resistance:** Two to three sessions per week. Three sets each of: bodyweight squats or goblet squats, Romanian deadlifts (or hip hinges with any available weight), rows (using resistance bands or a gym cable machine), push-up variations, and a plank hold. Full sessions take 30 to 40 minutes.
- **NEAT:** Minimum 7,000 steps per day measured by phone or watch. One to two movement breaks per work hour. Take stairs consistently.
- **Optional HIIT:** Replace one aerobic session per week with a 15- to 20-minute interval protocol: 30 seconds of effort (brisk walking up stairs, cycling hard, or jogging) followed by 60 to 90 seconds of easy movement. Repeat eight to ten times.

Advanced Plan—"Optimize and Progress"

Appropriate for: People with an established exercise habit who want to optimize their program for liver and metabolic health specifically.

- **Aerobic:** 150 to 200 minutes of moderate-intensity aerobic activity per week, distributed across four to five sessions.
- **Resistance:** Three sessions per week with progressive overload—gradually increasing resistance over time to continue stimulating muscle adaptation. Compound movements prioritized: squats, deadlifts, rows, presses. Two to three sets of eight to twelve repetitions per exercise at a challenging weight.
- **HIIT:** One to two sessions per week, separated by at least 48 hours of lower-intensity activity for recovery.
- **NEAT:** Target 7,000 to 10,000 steps per day—additional health gains decrease significantly after 7,000 steps per day, offering only slightly greater benefits such as improved glucose control.[118] Treat sedentary hours as a deliberate target to minimize, not a neutral baseline.
- **Recovery:** At this volume, adequate sleep and stress management become critical. Overtraining suppresses the immune system, elevates cortisol, and counteracts the metabolic benefits of exercise. One to two complete rest days per week are not optional—they are part of the program.

Overcoming Common Barriers

The barriers to consistent exercise are real and worth addressing directly, because dismissing them with generic motivational advice does not help anyone.

- **"I don't have time."** Thirty minutes of moderate exercise five days a week is 2.5 percent of your waking hours. Most people who say they don't have time have not yet made exercise a non-negotiable scheduling item—it gets treated as optional and displaced by other things. It helps to identify a specific, recurring time slot and protect it with the same firmness as a work meeting. If even thirty minutes is genuinely unavailable, fifteen minutes is meaningful. Three five-minute micro-sessions of bodyweight movement distributed through the day is meaningful. The dose-response curve rewards any movement over none.

- **"I'm too tired to exercise."** This is real and deserves empathy, particularly for people dealing with metabolic fatigue. The counterintuitive truth is that low-intensity exercise almost always improves energy levels rather than depleting them—the fatigue associated with inactivity is often broken by movement, not rest. Start with a ten-minute walk and gauge how you feel afterward. The most common report is that energy improves. If fatigue is severe and persistent, it warrants medical evaluation—it may reflect thyroid dysfunction, anemia, sleep apnea, or other contributing factors.

- **"I have joint pain or physical limitations."** Most forms of structured exercise can be modified for joint limitations. Walking in a pool (water walking) eliminates almost all joint impact while maintaining cardiovascular and metabolic benefit. Seated resistance exercises are effective for people with knee or ankle issues. Cycling—stationary or outdoor—is low-impact and highly effective for liver fat reduction. Work with your doctor or a physical therapist to identify the most appropriate starting point for your specific situation.

- **"I tried before and couldn't stick with it."** The most common reason exercise habits fail is mismatch between the program and the person's actual life. An exercise program designed for a twenty-five-year-old with a flexible schedule and no dependents will fail for a fifty-year-old parent with a demanding job—not because the fifty-year-old lacks discipline, but because the program was wrong for them. Design for your actual life: realistic schedule, realistic intensity, modalities you find at least tolerable, if not enjoyable. Enjoyment is a powerful predictor of adherence.

Start Here: Your First Two Weeks

If you are not currently exercising regularly, this is your minimum viable entry point. It is designed to be achievable regardless of fitness level, schedule, or available equipment.

Week 1

- Walk for 20 minutes every day. Any pace that elevates your breathing slightly. Outside, on a treadmill, around your building—location does not matter.
- Perform two sets of ten air squats twice during the workday (mid-morning and mid-afternoon). This takes less than two minutes total.
- Stand up and move briefly every hour during sedentary work periods.

Week 2

- Extend your daily walk to 25 to 30 minutes.

- Add a ten-minute bodyweight circuit three times this week: ten squats, ten push-ups (wall or floor), ten reverse lunges each leg, a 20-second plank. Rest one minute and repeat.
- Continue hourly movement breaks. Note your step count—aim to match or slightly exceed the previous day.

At the end of two weeks, you will have established a daily movement habit, introduced resistance training stimulus, and generated a cumulative exercise dose that the research associates with measurable improvements in liver fat markers within four to six weeks of continuation.

That is not a small thing. That is a liver that has begun to receive a different set of signals—and it will respond.

✦ ✦ ✦

Key Takeaways

- Exercise reduces liver fat, improves liver enzymes, and lowers liver inflammation independently of weight loss. You do not need to lose weight first to begin healing your liver through movement.
- The primary mechanisms are direct hepatic fat oxidation, improved muscle insulin sensitivity, myokine signaling from contracting muscles to the liver, and preferential visceral fat reduction.
- All three major exercise modalities—aerobic training, resistance training, and HIIT—produce meaningful liver benefit through partially distinct pathways. A combined program is optimal; any single modality consistently practiced is substantially better than none.

- Short bouts of bodyweight exercise—including air squats performed at regular intervals throughout the day—produce measurable cardiovascular, metabolic, and myokine benefits without requiring a gym or a long workout.
- NEAT—the accumulated physical movement of everyday life outside formal exercise—accounts for a major proportion of total activity-related energy expenditure and metabolic benefit. Moving more throughout the day matters as much as structured exercise.
- The single most important exercise principle: Something is always better than nothing. Design for your actual life, start where you are, and build consistency before building intensity.

Exercise and nutrition together form the most powerful combination available for liver repair. But for many people, the limiting factor is not what they eat or how much they move—it is what they weigh, and more specifically, where that weight is stored. Chapter 6 addresses the relationship between body weight, visceral fat, and the liver, including how to approach weight loss sustainably without the metabolic rebound that derails so many efforts.

CHAPTER 6

Weight Loss, Visceral Fat, and the Liver Connection

What the Scale Doesn't Tell You—and What Actually Matters

Two people step on the scale. Both weigh exactly 200 pounds. One has a healthy liver, good insulin sensitivity, and a relatively low metabolic risk profile. The other has significant fatty liver disease, insulin resistance, and elevated cardiovascular risk.

The number on the scale is identical. The metabolic reality could not be more different.

This chapter is about understanding why—and why the distinction matters enormously for how you approach weight loss as part of a liver health strategy. The goal is not a number on a scale. The goal is a specific type of fat loss, in a specific location, achieved through a specific approach that preserves the tissue that matters most for long-term metabolic health.

Get this right, and modest weight loss produces dramatic liver improvement. Get it wrong—lose weight too aggressively, or in a way that sacrifices muscle—and you can undermine the very metabolic machinery you are trying to repair.

Visceral Fat: The Fat That Actually Threatens Your Liver

Not all fat is created equal. The human body stores fat in two fundamentally different compartments, and they behave very differently from a metabolic standpoint.

Subcutaneous fat is the fat stored directly beneath the skin—the fat you can pinch on your abdomen, hips, thighs, and arms. It is metabolically relatively quiet. While excess subcutaneous fat is associated with higher overall body weight and some increase in metabolic risk, it does not drive liver disease directly. Some research even suggests that moderate subcutaneous fat in certain locations may have a neutral or mildly protective metabolic role.[119]

Visceral fat is the fat stored deep inside the abdominal cavity, wrapped around the internal organs—the intestines, kidneys, pancreas, and most importantly for our purposes, the liver. This fat is not quiet. It is one of the most metabolically active and harmful tissue types in the human body.

Visceral fat continuously releases a stream of inflammatory cytokines—particularly TNF-alpha, IL-6, and resistin—directly into the portal circulation that feeds the liver.[120] It releases free fatty acids at high rates, further overwhelming the liver's processing capacity.[121] It produces hormones that worsen insulin resistance throughout the body.[122] And unlike subcutaneous fat, visceral fat is highly responsive to the same insulin resistance and cortisol elevation that drive fatty liver disease—meaning MASLD and visceral fat accumulation tend to occur together and reinforce each other.[123]

Here is what makes this clinically important: A person can have significant visceral fat accumulation with a body weight that appears normal or only slightly elevated. This is sometimes called TOFI—thin outside, fat inside. Lean individuals with high visceral fat burden carry substantially elevated metabolic and liver disease risk, while overweight individuals with lower visceral fat relative to their total weight may have a more favorable metabolic profile than their BMI suggests.

This is why BMI alone is a poor predictor of MASLD risk and a poor guide to treatment response. Waist circumference—a simple proxy for visceral fat burden—is a more meaningful measurement. For most adults, a waist circumference above 35 inches in women and 40 inches in men is associated with meaningfully elevated visceral fat and metabolic risk. But even these thresholds are population averages, not individual verdicts.

> ***A More Useful Measurement Than the Scale.*** *Track your waist circumference at the level of your navel—measured first thing in the morning before eating, standing naturally without sucking in. This single measurement captures visceral fat changes more directly than body weight and tends to move in the right direction faster than the scale when lifestyle changes are working. Measure monthly, not weekly—short-term fluctuations are noise.*

The Good News: Visceral Fat Is Highly Responsive to Lifestyle

Of all the tissues in the body that accumulate pathologically in metabolic disease, visceral fat is among the most responsive to intervention. It is mobilized preferentially during caloric restriction, aerobic exercise, and periods of reduced insulin stimulation.[124] It disappears faster than subcutaneous fat when lifestyle changes are implemented—and the liver benefits are correspondingly rapid.

This preferential mobilization has a clear biological rationale. Visceral fat cells have a higher density of beta-adrenergic receptors—the receptor type that responds to the adrenaline and noradrenaline released during exercise and periods of reduced caloric intake.[125] They are, in a sense, primed to release their stored fat when the metabolic environment changes. The liver fat itself, which behaves similarly, is often the first depot to visibly reduce on imaging studies when dietary and exercise changes are implemented.

In other words, your belly fat is chemically different from the fat on the rest of your body. It is "wired" to be much more sensitive to your body's fat-burning signals. While the fat on your legs might be stubborn and slow to move, the fat deep in your belly is covered in "gas pedals" that respond instantly to exercise and movement. This is why when you start a new fitness routine, you often notice your waistline shrinking before you see changes anywhere else—your belly fat is simply more ready to be used as fuel.

The practical implication: Early feedback tends to come before the scale reflects it. Waist circumference often decreases noticeably within the first four to six weeks of consistent lifestyle change, even when total body weight has barely moved. Liver enzymes frequently normalize within eight to twelve weeks. These early signals are not cosmetic—they reflect genuine metabolic improvement happening precisely where it matters most.

Safe vs. Aggressive Weight Loss: Why the Rate Matters

It might seem intuitive that faster weight loss produces faster liver improvement. The evidence is more nuanced—and in some cases points in the opposite direction.

Rapid weight loss—typically defined as more than two pounds per week sustained over several weeks—carries a specific risk for people with fatty liver disease: It can temporarily worsen liver inflammation and accelerate fibrosis progression in some individuals.[126] The mechanism involves the rapid mobilization of large amounts of fatty acids from adipose tissue into circulation, overwhelming the liver's capacity to process them. Very low-calorie diets (under 800 calories per day) and extended fasting protocols can trigger this response, particularly in people with pre-existing MASH.

Rapid weight loss also dramatically increases the risk of gallstone formation.[127] The liver secretes bile to digest fat, and when fat intake drops sharply and weight loss is rapid, bile composition changes in ways that promote cholesterol crystallization in the gallbladder. Gallstones develop in a significant proportion of people who lose weight very rapidly—a complication that can require surgical intervention and is entirely avoidable with a more moderate pace.

The evidence-based target for safe, effective weight loss in fatty liver disease is 0.5 to 1 kilogram per week—approximately one to two pounds. At this rate, fat loss is predominantly from adipose tissue (including visceral fat) rather than muscle. Liver fat clears steadily. The risk of gallstone formation is substantially lower. And the hormonal and metabolic adaptations to weight loss are less severe, making long-term maintenance more achievable.

This pace requires a modest, sustainable caloric deficit—roughly 500 calories per day below maintenance, achievable through a combination of improved food quality, reduced portion size, and increased physical activity. It does not require extreme restriction or rigid calorie counting for most people. When food quality improves meaningfully, caloric intake often falls naturally into a moderate deficit as appetite regulation normalizes.

Plateau Physiology: Why Weight Loss Stalls and What to Do About It

Almost everyone who pursues intentional weight loss encounters a plateau—a period during which weight loss slows dramatically or stops entirely despite continued effort. For many people, this is the point where discouragement sets in and the program collapses. Understanding why plateaus occur makes them far less demoralizing, and far more navigable.

The primary driver of weight loss plateaus is metabolic adaptation. When caloric intake is reduced and body weight decreases, the body responds by reducing its total energy expenditure—a phenomenon researchers call adaptive thermogenesis. This is not a failure of willpower or a character flaw. It is a predictable, biologically programmed response to what the body interprets as a food scarcity event.

Several specific adaptations occur. Resting metabolic rate decreases—partly because a smaller body simply requires fewer calories to maintain, and partly because of active metabolic suppression beyond what body composition changes alone would predict. Non-exercise activity thermogenesis (NEAT) decreases unconsciously—people move slightly less throughout the day, fidget less, and expend less energy in routine activities without realizing it. Appetite-stimulating hormones like ghrelin rise. Satiety hormones like leptin fall. The body becomes a more efficient energy conservation machine, precisely when you are trying to create a deficit.

This adaptation does not mean progress has stopped or that further improvement is impossible. It means the initial approach needs recalibration.

Practical Strategies for Breaking Through a Plateau

- **Reassess caloric intake honestly:** As body weight decreases, caloric maintenance needs decrease as well. A deficit that produced weight loss at 220 pounds may be maintenance at 195 pounds. Recalculating your target intake based on current body weight—rather than the weight you started at—can restart progress.
- **Increase exercise volume or intensity:** Adding ten to fifteen minutes to aerobic sessions, introducing HIIT (high-intensity interval training), or adding a resistance training session increases energy expenditure and stimulates

metabolic adaptations that partially counteract the efficiency gains of adaptation.

- **Prioritize protein:** Higher protein intake preserves muscle mass during weight loss, which in turn preserves resting metabolic rate. Ensuring adequate protein (1.2 to 1.6 g/kg/day) at a plateau helps maintain the metabolic engine.
- **Incorporate diet breaks strategically:** Short periods of eating at caloric maintenance—one to two weeks—can partially reset leptin levels, reduce the severity of metabolic adaptation, and make the subsequent return to a deficit more effective. This is not the same as abandoning the program. It is a planned recalibration.
- **Improve sleep and stress management:** Cortisol elevation from chronic stress and sleep deprivation directly impairs fat mobilization and promotes fat storage, particularly in the visceral compartment. Addressing these factors during a plateau often produces renewed progress even without further dietary changes.

Perhaps most importantly: Remember that a weight loss plateau does not mean a liver health plateau. During periods when the scale is not moving, the liver may still be improving—enzyme levels normalizing, inflammation reducing, fat clearing from hepatic tissue. The liver does not require continuous weight loss to continue healing. It requires a consistently favorable metabolic environment, which you may already be providing.

Body Contouring Procedures: What They Can and Cannot Do

Procedures like CoolSculpting (cryolipolysis)—which use controlled cooling to selectively destroy subcutaneous fat cells in targeted areas—have become popular as a complement to lifestyle-based weight loss. They are worth addressing directly, because people with fatty liver disease sometimes inquire about them in the context of their overall management strategy.

The honest answer is this: Body contouring procedures target subcutaneous fat—the fat beneath the skin. They have no meaningful effect on visceral fat, the fat most directly relevant to liver disease and metabolic health. CoolSculpting can reduce the volume of a subcutaneous fat deposit in a localized area, but it does not improve insulin sensitivity, reduce liver fat, lower inflammatory cytokines, or address any of the root causes of MASLD.

For people who have already achieved meaningful lifestyle-based improvements and are managing a residual subcutaneous fat deposit that is cosmetically concerning to them, body contouring procedures may have a role. But they belong, if at all, at the end of a successful lifestyle program—not as a substitute for one, and not as a primary strategy for someone still working to improve their metabolic health.

One important safety consideration: CoolSculpting and similar procedures are elective cosmetic interventions with their own risk profiles, including rare but documented complications such as paradoxical adipose hyperplasia—a condition in which the treated area actually increases in size rather than decreasing. For anyone with active liver disease, elective procedures should be discussed with the hepatologist managing their care before proceeding.

Bariatric Surgery: When Lifestyle Is Not Enough

For a subset of people with fatty liver disease—particularly those with severe obesity (BMI above 40, or above 35 with significant metabolic comorbidities) who have not achieved adequate results through sustained lifestyle intervention—bariatric surgery represents a legitimate and evidence-supported option.

The results of bariatric surgery on fatty liver disease are among the most dramatic in the field. Studies following individuals after Roux-en-Y gastric bypass and sleeve gastrectomy have documented resolution of MASH in 85 to 90 percent of patients, significant fibrosis regression in over 70 percent, and near-complete normalization of liver histology in many cases.[128] These are outcomes that no lifestyle program or medication can reliably match in severe disease.

The mechanisms extend well beyond the caloric restriction that follows the procedure. Bariatric surgery produces profound hormonal changes—alterations in GLP-1, PYY, ghrelin, and bile acid metabolism—that improve insulin sensitivity, reduce appetite, and directly benefit liver metabolism in ways that persist independently of the weight loss itself. This hormonal remodeling is one reason why liver improvement after bariatric surgery often begins within days of the procedure, before significant weight loss has occurred.

Bariatric surgery is not without significant risk. Surgery complications, nutritional deficiencies (particularly in B vitamins, iron, calcium, and fat-soluble vitamins), dumping syndrome, psychological adjustment challenges, and the need for lifelong dietary modification and nutritional monitoring are all real considerations. It is major surgery, and it requires a committed, well-supported patient who understands what the procedure involves and what the long-term obligations are.

The appropriate context for bariatric surgery in fatty liver disease is a conversation between a patient and a multidisciplinary care team—typically including a hepatologist, a bariatric surgeon, a dietitian, a lifestyle coach, and a psychologist—after lifestyle intervention has been genuinely and consistently attempted. It is a powerful option for the right person. It is not a shortcut, and it is not appropriate as a first-line response to a diagnosis of early-stage fatty liver disease in someone who has not yet engaged seriously with lifestyle change.

Maintaining Results: The Phase Most Plans Ignore

Most weight loss programs are designed to get people to a goal. Very few are designed for what comes after—and this is where the research on long-term outcomes is most sobering.

Studies tracking weight loss outcomes over five years consistently show that the majority of lost weight is regained within two to five years in most people.[129] The biological mechanisms driving this are the same metabolic adaptations described in the plateau section—lower resting metabolic rate, altered appetite hormones, unconscious reduction in NEAT—that persist long after active weight loss ends. The body defends its prior weight setpoint with impressive persistence.

For liver health specifically, weight regain is not simply a cosmetic or fitness setback. Studies have shown that weight regain after liver fat reduction is associated with rapid return of hepatic steatosis, sometimes to levels worse than the original baseline. The liver is responsive in both directions.

Long-term maintenance requires a fundamentally different approach than the weight loss phase—not because the behaviors are different, but because the motivation structure needs to shift. During weight loss, progress itself provides feedback and motivation. During maintenance, there is no visible progress—only the absence of regression. This requires a different psychological orientation: the recognition that the lifestyle behaviors that produced improvement are not a temporary program with a finish line. They are the new normal.

What Maintenance Actually Looks Like

The research on long-term weight maintenance identifies a consistent set of behaviors in people who successfully keep weight off for five or more years. These are not surprising, but they are specific enough to be actionable.

- **Consistent physical activity:** Long-term maintainers consistently engage in higher levels of physical activity than the general population—typically 60 or more minutes of moderate activity most days. This higher activity level compensates for the reduced resting metabolic rate that accompanies weight loss and creates the ongoing metabolic environment that keeps the liver healthy. Resistance training is particularly valuable for maintaining muscle mass and resting metabolism during the maintenance phase.
- **Continued dietary vigilance (without rigidity):** Successful maintainers do not eat perfectly all the time, but they maintain consistent awareness of their food choices and return quickly to their baseline after deviations. The "monitoring" does not have to be formal calorie counting—it can be as simple as maintaining awareness of when eating has drifted toward old patterns and course-correcting promptly.
- **Regular self-monitoring:** Weighing regularly—not obsessively, but consistently—and scheduling periodic lab checks provides early warning if metabolic health is slipping. A five-pound gain caught early is far easier to address than a twenty-pound gain noticed after months of denial.
- **Consistent sleep and stress management:** The hormonal environment created by adequate sleep and managed stress directly supports weight maintenance by keeping cortisol, ghrelin, and leptin in favorable ranges. These behaviors, which may have started as part of a liver health program, need to persist as permanent features of a healthy life.

- **Identity shift:** Perhaps the most powerful predictor of long-term success is whether a person comes to see their healthy behaviors as part of who they are rather than as a program they are following. "I eat this way because I value my health" is a more durable behavioral driver than "I am currently on a diet." This shift does not happen through willpower—it happens through the accumulation of consistent actions over time that gradually redefine your sense of what normal looks and feels like.

Start Here: Your Weight Loss Strategy Checklist

Set the Right Goal

- Target 0.5 to 1 kilogram (1.1 to 2.2 pounds) per week as a safe, sustainable pace
- Measure waist circumference monthly as a more meaningful metric than daily scale weight
- Set an early milestone: a five percent reduction in body weight, at which point liver fat improvements are typically already measurable

Protect Your Muscle

- Maintain protein intake at 1.2 to 1.6 g/kg of body weight throughout the weight loss phase
- Continue resistance training at least twice per week during caloric restriction—muscle is not an acceptable casualty of weight loss
- Avoid extreme caloric restriction (under 1,200 calories/day for women, 1,500 for men) without medical supervision

Prepare for the Plateau

- Expect a slowdown between weeks six and twelve—this is normal physiology, not failure
- When the plateau arrives, recalculate your caloric target based on your current weight rather than your starting weight
- Consider a one-to-two-week maintenance break before resuming a deficit

Build for Maintenance from the Start

- Practice the eating pattern and exercise habits you intend to maintain permanently, not a temporary extreme version
- Schedule a six-month and twelve-month lab check to confirm that metabolic markers are holding
- Treat a five-pound regain as an early warning signal that warrants prompt attention, not a reason for shame or catastrophizing

✦ ✦ ✦

Key Takeaways

- Visceral fat—not subcutaneous fat—is the primary fat depot driving liver inflammation and metabolic dysfunction. Waist circumference is a more clinically meaningful measurement than scale weight for tracking liver-relevant fat loss.
- Visceral fat is highly responsive to lifestyle intervention and is preferentially mobilized during aerobic exercise and modest caloric restriction. Liver fat clears rapidly as visceral fat declines—often faster than the scale reflects.

- Safe, effective weight loss for fatty liver disease targets 0.5 to 1 kilogram per week. Faster rates risk temporary worsening of liver inflammation, gallstone formation, and muscle loss that undermines long-term metabolic health.
- Weight loss plateaus are driven by predictable metabolic adaptations, not failure. They are navigable with recalibration of caloric targets, increased exercise, strategic diet breaks, and attention to sleep and stress.
- Body contouring procedures like CoolSculpting target subcutaneous fat only and have no meaningful effect on the visceral fat or metabolic dysfunction driving fatty liver disease.
- Bariatric surgery produces dramatic, evidence-supported improvements in advanced fatty liver disease for appropriate candidates—but is not a first-line response and requires a comprehensive multidisciplinary evaluation.
- Long-term maintenance requires a permanent lifestyle shift, not a temporary program. The behaviors that produce improvement need to become the new normal—supported by continued activity, consistent monitoring, and an identity that embraces health rather than tolerates restriction.

Nutrition, exercise, and weight management form the core triad of fatty liver disease reversal. But two additional lifestyle factors can silently undermine every other effort if left unaddressed: sleep and stress. Chapter 7 examines how sleep deprivation and chronic stress directly drive liver fat accumulation through hormonal pathways—and provides practical, evidence-grounded tools for addressing both.

CHAPTER 7

Sleep, Stress, and Hormonal Balance

The Hidden Drivers That Undermine Everything Else

Here is a scenario that plays out more often than most people realize. Someone commits seriously to improving their liver health. They overhaul their diet, cut out sugar-sweetened beverages, start exercising regularly. After four to six weeks, their energy is better, their clothes fit differently, and they are cautiously optimistic.

Then progress stalls. Liver enzymes that were trending down level off. Weight loss slows. Cravings return with unusual intensity. The discipline that felt sustainable a few weeks ago starts fraying. Something is working against them.

In a significant proportion of cases, that something is sleep deprivation and unmanaged chronic stress. Not as background noise, but as active biological forces that directly counteract the improvements being made elsewhere. You can eat well, move regularly, and still be undermining your liver's ability to heal if you are sleeping five or six hours a night and running on sustained cortisol.

This chapter addresses two of the most underappreciated drivers of fatty liver disease—and two of the most underutilized levers for reversing it. The science is unambiguous. The practical tools are accessible. And for many people, addressing sleep and stress produces metabolic improvements that dietary and exercise changes alone have been unable to deliver.

Sleep Deprivation and the Liver: A Direct Biological Connection

Sleep is not rest. It is an active, metabolically essential process during which the body carries out maintenance and repair that simply cannot be accomplished while awake. The liver, in particular, has a carefully orchestrated overnight program: clearing metabolic waste, resetting insulin signaling, modulating inflammatory activity, and performing the cellular housekeeping that keeps it functional during the day.[130]

When sleep is chronically insufficient—most research defines this as consistently fewer than seven hours per night—this overnight program is interrupted.[131] The consequences for metabolic health accumulate quickly and are measurable within days of sleep restriction.

A landmark study from the University of Chicago found that just one week of sleep restriction to five to six hours per night reduced insulin sensitivity by approximately 25 percent in otherwise healthy young adults.[132] This is a degree of insulin resistance comparable to what would take months of poor diet and physical inactivity to produce through lifestyle alone—achieved in a single week by simply not sleeping enough.

The mechanism involves multiple hormonal pathways operating simultaneously. When sleep is cut short, cortisol levels rise and remain elevated into the following day. Growth hormone secretion—

which normally peaks during deep sleep and plays a critical role in fat metabolism and tissue repair—is blunted. The sympathetic nervous system remains in a low-grade activated state, keeping the body in a metabolic posture more suited to threat response than to healing.

For the liver specifically, sleep deprivation elevates circulating free fatty acids, increases hepatic glucose production (the liver releases more glucose into the blood even when blood sugar is already adequate), and activates the inflammatory pathways most closely associated with the progression from simple steatosis to MASH. Research directly linking short sleep duration to higher rates of fatty liver disease and worse disease severity now spans multiple large population studies, including data from the UK Biobank and the NHANES survey.

The Appetite Disruption Problem

Sleep deprivation's effect on appetite is one of the most robustly documented and practically significant findings in metabolic research—and it is directly relevant to anyone trying to improve their liver health through dietary change.

After a night of insufficient sleep, ghrelin—the hormone that signals hunger and drives food-seeking behavior—rises measurably.[133] Leptin—the hormone that signals satiety and suppresses appetite—falls.[134] The result is a predictable, reliable drive toward increased caloric intake on the following day. Studies have consistently found that sleep-deprived individuals consume 300 to 500 additional calories per day compared to when they are adequately rested—without any change in their conscious dietary intentions.[135,136,137]

The food choices made under sleep deprivation are also specifically skewed toward high-carbohydrate, high-sugar, and ultra-processed options.[138] The prefrontal cortex—the brain region responsible for impulse control and long-term decision-making—is disproportionately impaired by sleep loss.[139] The reward circuits that drive cravings for palatable, calorie-dense food are relatively spared and actually become hyperresponsive. The biological deck is stacked against good food choices when you are tired.

Here is the practical implication: If you are consistently sleeping fewer than seven hours and struggling with dietary adherence—experiencing intense cravings, finding it difficult to eat the way you intend—sleep deprivation may be the primary obstacle, not lack of motivation or willpower. Fixing the sleep may fix the adherence problem in ways that no amount of dietary discipline can.

Circadian Rhythm and Liver Metabolism: The Body Clock Connection

Every cell in the human body contains a molecular clock—a set of genes that cycle through activation and suppression on roughly a 24-hour rhythm, coordinating the timing of metabolic processes with the external light-dark cycle.[140] The liver has one of the most sophisticated peripheral clocks in the body, and a remarkable proportion of its gene activity—estimated at 15 to 20 percent of the liver's entire genome—follows a circadian pattern.[141]

What this means practically is that the liver is not equally capable at all hours. It is best equipped to process carbohydrates, manage insulin signaling, and perform active metabolic work during daylight hours. Its detoxification and repair programs run predominantly during the night. These programs are not interchangeable—eating a large meal at 10 PM does not produce the same metabolic response as eating the same meal at noon, even if the calories and macronutrients are identical.

As established in Chapter 2, people with fatty liver disease show a specific nighttime metabolic dysfunction—reduced insulin secretion and higher insulin clearance during overnight hours—that persists even after weight loss. The liver's circadian clock is disrupted in MASLD, and this disruption is now understood to be a core feature of the disease rather than simply a consequence of it.

Circadian misalignment—when your actual schedule of eating, light exposure, activity, and sleep is misaligned with your biological clock—amplifies every aspect of this dysfunction. Shift workers have some of the highest rates of metabolic syndrome and fatty liver disease of any occupational group.[142,143] People who eat the majority of their calories in the evening, who use bright screens late at night, and who have highly variable sleep schedules show consistently worse metabolic profiles than those who align their behavior with their biological clock.[144]

The good news is that circadian alignment is largely within your control. The specific behavioral strategies for realigning your body clock are among the most practical and impactful tools in this chapter.

Chronic Stress, Cortisol, and Fat Storage

The relationship between stress and liver disease is not metaphorical. It is physiological, direct, and mediated by one of the most powerful hormones in the human body.

Cortisol is produced by the adrenal glands in response to any perceived threat or stressor—physical danger, work pressure, financial anxiety, relationship conflict, even the physiological stress of sleep deprivation. In short bursts, cortisol is adaptive and life-sustaining. It mobilizes energy, sharpens focus, suppresses nonessential functions, and prepares the body for action.

Chronic stress means chronic cortisol elevation—and sustained high cortisol is profoundly damaging to metabolic health.[145] It promotes insulin resistance directly by interfering with insulin receptor signaling in liver and muscle cells. It drives the preferential accumulation of visceral fat by activating glucocorticoid receptors in abdominal adipose tissue, which respond to cortisol by storing fat rather than releasing it. It stimulates the liver to produce and release glucose even when blood sugar is already adequate—a process called hepatic gluconeogenesis—creating a persistent background elevation in blood sugar and insulin demand.

Cortisol also activates the inflammatory pathways most directly implicated in the progression of fatty liver disease.[146] High cortisol increases the production of TNF-alpha and IL-6—the same inflammatory cytokines released by visceral fat that drive hepatic inflammation in MASLD.[147] Chronic stress and high visceral fat thus operate through overlapping inflammatory channels, compounding each other's damage to the liver.

Research published in the journal *Hepatology* found that perceived stress scores were independently associated with higher ALT levels and worse liver histology (structure and organization, including cells, tissues, and functional units) in MASLD patients—after controlling for diet, exercise, body weight, and alcohol intake.[148] Stress is not merely undermining your motivation to make good choices. It is independently worsening your liver disease through a hormonal pathway that operates whether or not you are aware of it.

The HPA Axis: Why Chronic Stress Is Self-Perpetuating

The hypothalamic-pituitary-adrenal (HPA) axis is the biological circuit that governs the stress response. Under healthy conditions, it operates with a self-regulating feedback loop: A stressor triggers cortisol release, cortisol does its job, and then inhibitory signals bring cortisol back down. The system resets.

Under chronic stress, this feedback loop becomes dysregulated. The inhibitory signals weaken. Cortisol stays elevated at baseline. The threshold for triggering another stress response drops, meaning smaller provocations produce larger responses. The system becomes sensitized—progressively less capable of fully returning to a calm, recovery-oriented state.

This sensitization has direct implications for liver health. Each stress response further impairs insulin sensitivity. Disrupted sleep—itself a cortisol-elevating stressor—feeds back into the HPA axis, raising baseline cortisol further. Elevated cortisol promotes cravings for high-sugar, high-fat foods, which when consumed drive more insulin resistance and liver fat. The loop closes on itself, and breaking it requires deliberate, sustained intervention at multiple points simultaneously.

This is not a reason for alarm—it is a reason for strategy. The parasympathetic nervous system (the body's rest-and-digest counterpart to the stress response) can be activated deliberately, and with practice, more reliably. Every evidence-based stress reduction tool works through the same basic mechanism: activating the parasympathetic system, lowering cortisol, and interrupting the self-reinforcing stress loop.

Practical Sleep Optimization: A Protocol That Works

Sleep quality and quantity are improvable with behavioral intervention for most people. The following protocol is grounded in sleep medicine research and structured around the factors with the strongest evidence for improving sleep in metabolically unhealthy adults.

Establish a Consistent Sleep-Wake Schedule

The single most important sleep behavior is consistency. Going to bed and waking at the same time every day—including weekends—anchors your circadian clock and improves sleep quality more reliably than any other single intervention. Weekend sleep schedule drift of more than sixty to ninety minutes is associated with measurably worse metabolic markers through a phenomenon called social jetlag.

Choose a wake time you can maintain seven days a week and work backwards from it to determine your target bedtime. Protect both ends of the window with the same firmness as a professional commitment.

Manage Light Exposure Strategically

Light is the primary signal that sets your circadian clock. Morning bright light exposure—ideally natural sunlight within the first thirty to sixty minutes of waking—suppresses residual melatonin, raises cortisol appropriately at the start of the day, and anchors the timing of your entire biological clock. This morning cortisol rise, called the cortisol awakening response, is actually healthy and sets the rhythm for the day.

Evening light exposure from screens, overhead lighting, and devices emits blue-spectrum wavelengths that suppress melatonin production and signal the brain that it is still daytime. Reducing screen brightness, using blue-light filtering settings after 8 PM, switching to warmer-spectrum lighting in the evening, and avoiding bright overhead lights in the two hours before bed all support the natural melatonin rise that prepares the body for sleep.

This is not about eliminating evening screen use entirely—that is an unrealistic standard for most people. It is about reducing the blue-light signal sufficiently that melatonin can begin rising on schedule.

A Note on Your Light Bulbs

Most people manage their evening light exposure by dimming screens and reaching for blue-light filter settings—and that is a worthwhile start. What fewer people consider is the light coming from the bulbs in their ceiling fixtures, lamps, and overhead lighting.

Modern LED bulbs have largely replaced incandescent lighting in most homes due to their greater energy-efficiency and longer life. But the dominant color spectrum of standard LED bulbs skews heavily toward the blue-white range—a wavelength profile that is efficient for visibility but poorly suited for the hours when your brain needs to begin its transition toward sleep. Incandescent bulbs, for all their inefficiency, emitted a warmer, amber-toned light that more closely resembled firelight and was inherently less disruptive to melatonin production. Standard cool-white or daylight LED bulbs in the evening send essentially the same circadian signal as midday sunlight: stay awake.

The fix is straightforward and inexpensive. LED bulbs are now manufactured across a wide range of color temperatures, measured in Kelvin. Bulbs rated at 2,700K or below emit a warm, amber-toned light that is far less melatonin-suppressing than the 4,000K to 6,500K cool-white and daylight bulbs common in most fixtures.

Swapping the bulbs in your bedroom, living room, and any other rooms you use in the two hours before bed to warm-white LEDs (look for 2,700K or "soft white" on the packaging; some are 1,400 to 1,800 amber bulbs) is a one-time, low-cost environmental change that supports circadian alignment every night without any ongoing effort or discipline.

For those who want to go further, smart bulbs with tunable color temperature—such as those in the Philips Hue or LIFX product lines—can be programmed to automatically shift from cooler, higher-energy light during the day to warm amber tones in the evening, essentially automating the circadian light signal your home produces around the clock. This is the closest most people will get to the natural light environment the human circadian system evolved with: bright and blue-rich during the day, warm and dim as the sun goes down.

The investment of replacing a handful of bulbs is modest. The cumulative effect on melatonin timing, sleep onset, and sleep quality—night after night, year after year—is not.

Create a Thermal and Environmental Cue for Sleep

Core body temperature drops during sleep, and this drop is both a signal and a facilitator of sleep onset. A bedroom kept slightly cool—between 65 and 68 degrees Fahrenheit for most people—supports this natural thermal decline. A warm bath or shower thirty to sixty minutes before bed paradoxically accelerates sleep onset by drawing blood to the skin surface, facilitating the core temperature drop that signals sleep readiness.

Darkness and quietness in the sleep environment are foundational but worth reaffirming. Blackout curtains or a sleep mask eliminate light intrusion. Consistent white noise or earplugs mitigate sound disruption. These environmental factors consistently improve both sleep onset time and sleep continuity in research settings.

Address the Most Common Sleep Disruptors

- **Alcohol:** Alcohol may help with initial sleep onset but reliably fragments sleep in the second half of the night by suppressing REM sleep and disrupting sleep architecture. For people with fatty liver disease, its metabolic harms compound the sleep disruption—a double reason to reduce or eliminate evening alcohol.
- **Caffeine:** Caffeine has a half-life of approximately five to six hours in most adults, meaning that a coffee consumed at 3 PM still has half its caffeine active at 8 PM. For people who are sensitive to caffeine or who sleep poorly, cutting the caffeine window to before noon and observing whether sleep quality improves is a worthwhile experiment.
- **Late eating:** Eating within two to three hours of bedtime elevates insulin, raises core body temperature, and activates digestive processes that compete with the liver's overnight repair program. This is the same circadian rationale established in Chapter 2—late eating is a direct stressor on the liver's night-shift function.
- **Obstructive sleep apnea:** This is worth addressing directly and without understatement. Obstructive sleep apnea (OSA)—a condition in which the airway repeatedly collapses during sleep, causing brief awakenings and oxygen desaturations—is independently associated with worse fatty liver disease, accelerated fibrosis, and higher cardiovascular

risk.[149,150,151] It is also dramatically underdiagnosed. If you snore loudly, wake feeling unrefreshed despite adequate hours in bed, or have been told you stop breathing during sleep, evaluation by a sleep specialist is warranted. Treating OSA with CPAP, mouthpiece designed to help manage OSA, or other interventions consistently improves metabolic markers, liver enzymes, and sleep quality in studies of people with MASLD.[152,153]

Evidence-Based Stress Reduction: Tools That Work

Stress management is often dismissed as soft—a nice idea that doesn't belong in the same conversation as clinical interventions. The evidence does not support this dismissal. Structured stress reduction practices produce measurable reductions in cortisol, improvements in insulin sensitivity, and improvements in liver enzyme levels in clinical studies.[154]

The goal is not the elimination of stress—that is neither possible nor desirable. The goal is developing a practiced, reliable capacity to activate the parasympathetic nervous system and allow the body to recover from stress. Recovery is the operative word. The biological damage from chronic stress comes not from stress itself but from insufficient recovery. A stressed body that consistently recovers is metabolically very different from a stressed body that never does.

Breathing Practices

Controlled breathing is the fastest, most accessible tool for activating the parasympathetic nervous system. The vagus nerve—the primary conduit of the parasympathetic system—is directly stimulated by slow, deep exhalations. Extended exhale breathing, where the exhale is longer than the inhale, reliably lowers heart rate, reduces cortisol, and shifts the nervous system toward a recovery state within minutes.

The most extensively studied protocol is the 4-7-8 breath: inhale for four counts, hold for seven, exhale slowly for eight. Three to five cycles of this pattern produce a measurable parasympathetic shift. Box breathing—four counts in, four counts hold, four counts out, four counts hold—is used by military personnel and emergency responders for rapid stress regulation and is equally accessible.

The practical strategy: two to five minutes of controlled breathing twice daily—once in the morning before high-stress activity and once before sleep—produces cumulative cortisol-lowering effects that are detectable over weeks of consistent practice. This is a two-to-five-minute investment. The barrier is low; the evidence is real.

Mindfulness and Meditation

Mindfulness-based stress reduction (MBSR) has been studied more extensively than any other behavioral stress intervention. A meta-analysis of over 200 controlled trials found consistent reductions in cortisol, inflammatory markers, blood pressure, and psychological stress scores across diverse populations.[155] For MASLD specifically, mindfulness-based interventions have been shown to improve dietary adherence, reduce emotional eating, lower ALT levels, and improve quality of life in pilot trials.[156,157]

Formal meditation practice—even ten to fifteen minutes daily—produces these benefits over eight to twelve weeks of consistent practice. Guided meditation apps (Headspace, Calm, Insight Timer, and others) provide structured, progressive programs that are accessible to beginners without any prior experience or special training.

Informal mindfulness—bringing deliberate, nonjudgmental attention to routine activities like eating, walking, or even washing dishes—is less well-studied but mechanistically plausible and practically valuable for people who find formal sitting meditation difficult to sustain.

Nature Exposure

Time spent in natural environments—parks, forests, gardens, bodies of water, even tree-lined streets—produces measurable reductions in cortisol, blood pressure, heart rate, and self-reported stress. Japanese research on "forest bathing" (*shinrin-yoku*) has documented significant reductions in salivary cortisol after as little as twenty minutes in a forested environment.[158]

The mechanisms are not fully understood but appear to involve a combination of reduced cognitive load (natural environments require less directed attention than urban environments), exposure to phytoncides (therapeutic volatile compounds released by trees that have measurable immunological effects when inhaled), and activation of the parasympathetic nervous system through engagement of the visual and auditory systems with nonthreatening sensory input.

Twenty to thirty minutes in a natural environment two to three times per week is sufficient to produce measurable stress reduction effects in research settings. This does not require access to wilderness. A local park, a garden, or a walk along a river or lakefront qualifies. Crucially, nature exposure is most effective when devices are set aside—the cortisol-lowering benefit of a forest walk is substantially diminished when the walk is spent checking email.

Social Connection and Support

Chronic loneliness and social isolation activate the HPA axis and maintain elevated baseline cortisol as reliably as any external stressor.[159] The neuroscience is clear: The human stress system was calibrated in an environment where social disconnection was genuinely dangerous. The body treats sustained isolation as a threat, with all the corresponding hormonal consequences.

Quality social connection—time with people whose company is genuinely restorative, not merely obligatory—activates the release of oxytocin, which directly suppresses cortisol and lowers the HPA axis setpoint. For people managing a chronic health condition, the social support dimension of the recovery environment is not peripheral. It is, for many people, one of the most powerful variables in their long-term outcomes.

This does not require a large social network or dramatic social changes. Research suggests that the quality of a small number of close relationships is more protective than a large number of superficial ones.[160] Identifying the relationships in your life that are genuinely restorative and investing in them—rather than allowing them to atrophy in the busy-ness of daily life—is a legitimate and evidence-supported liver health strategy.

Hormonal Balance: The Broader Picture

Sleep, stress, and circadian rhythm all intersect with a wider hormonal ecosystem that influences liver health. Two hormonal considerations beyond cortisol deserve brief attention here, as they frequently arise in the context of MASLD.

Thyroid Function

Hypothyroidism—underactive thyroid function—is significantly more common in people with fatty liver disease than in the general population, and the relationship is bidirectional.[161] Low thyroid hormone impairs the liver's ability to export and oxidize fat, worsens insulin resistance, promotes weight gain, and causes the kind of fatigue that undermines every other lifestyle intervention. Thyroid dysfunction is also frequently underdiagnosed because standard TSH testing does not capture the full picture of thyroid function.

If you are experiencing persistent fatigue, cold intolerance, unexplained weight gain, hair thinning, or difficulty losing weight despite genuine lifestyle effort, thyroid evaluation is worth requesting from your doctor—including free T3 and free T4 levels, thyroid antibodies, and rT3, not just TSH. Optimizing thyroid function, where dysfunction exists, is a meaningful lever for metabolic and liver health that no amount of dietary discipline can substitute for.

Sex Hormones

Testosterone in men and estrogen in women both play regulatory roles in liver fat metabolism, and their decline with age is one reason that fatty liver disease risk increases significantly in middle age and beyond.[162]

In men, low testosterone is independently associated with higher visceral fat, worse insulin sensitivity, and elevated liver fat. The relationship appears to be bidirectional—low testosterone promotes metabolic dysfunction, and metabolic dysfunction (particularly high visceral fat) accelerates testosterone decline through aromatization of testosterone to estrogen in adipose tissue.

In women, the menopause transition is associated with a significant shift in fat distribution from subcutaneous to visceral, worsening insulin resistance, and increased liver fat accumulation. The hormonal environment of perimenopause and post-menopause increases MASLD risk, which partly explains why women, who have historically lower rates of fatty liver disease than men in younger adulthood, approach equivalent rates in their fifties and sixties.

These hormonal considerations are not amenable to simple lifestyle fixes, but they are worth discussing with a healthcare provider if they are likely contributors to your metabolic picture. Lifestyle optimization—particularly adequate sleep, stress management, resistance training, and visceral fat reduction—supports favorable hormonal balance and partly mitigates these age-related shifts.

Start Here: Your Sleep and Stress Reset Protocol

The following is a minimum viable protocol for improving sleep and managing stress over a four-week period. It is designed to be added to an existing dietary and exercise program rather than replacing it.

Week 1 – Establish the Foundation

- Set a fixed wake time and maintain it every day, including weekends. Choose a time you can realistically sustain.
- Get outside for natural light exposure within the first hour of waking each morning—even five to ten minutes on a clear day is meaningful.
- Move your last meal to at least two hours before bedtime. Three hours is better.
- Dim overhead lights and reduce screen brightness after 9 PM.

Week 2 – Add Active Recovery

- Begin a two-minute controlled breathing practice before bed each night: four counts in, hold briefly, six to eight counts out. Repeat five times.
- Schedule one twenty-minute nature exposure this week—a park walk, time in a garden, any natural setting with devices set aside.
- Identify and address the most significant sleep disruptor in your current routine: late caffeine, alcohol, late eating, or device use. Target one change this week.

Week 3 – Build Stress Resilience

- Add a morning breathing practice in addition to the evening one. Two minutes of controlled breathing within the first thirty minutes of waking sets the hormonal tone for the day.
- Begin a ten-minute guided meditation practice three times this week. Use a guided app if you are new to meditation—do not attempt to figure it out without structure.
- Schedule at least one genuinely restorative social interaction this week. Quality over quantity.

Week 4 – Consolidate and Assess

- Evaluate your average sleep duration. Are you consistently reaching seven to eight hours? If not, identify the specific barrier: difficulty falling asleep, waking in the night, or insufficient time budgeted for sleep.
- Note any changes in morning energy, afternoon cravings, or overall dietary adherence. Many people report that these improve noticeably after three to four weeks of sleep optimization—before any other changes are made.

- If you suspect obstructive sleep apnea—loud snoring, morning headaches, waking unrefreshed—discuss evaluation with your doctor this month.

> ***The Compounding Effect.*** *Better sleep reduces cortisol. Lower cortisol improves insulin sensitivity. Better insulin sensitivity reduces cravings for high-sugar foods. Fewer cravings improve dietary adherence. Better diet improves sleep quality. The system works in both directions. The goal is to make as many of these cycles run in the positive direction simultaneously—and sleep is often the linchpin that holds the rest of the strategy together.*

Key Takeaways

- Sleep deprivation is an active metabolic stressor that reduces insulin sensitivity by up to 25 percent within a week, elevates cortisol, disrupts appetite hormones, and directly worsens the inflammatory and metabolic environment driving fatty liver disease.
- The liver operates on a circadian clock. Disrupting the alignment of eating, light exposure, activity, and sleep with the biological clock amplifies the nighttime metabolic dysfunction characteristic of MASLD—and aligning behavior with the clock is one of the most underutilized tools for liver health.
- Chronic stress drives fatty liver disease through a direct hormonal pathway: Cortisol promotes insulin resistance, visceral fat accumulation, hepatic glucose overproduction, and liver inflammation independently of diet or exercise behavior.

- The HPA axis becomes sensitized under chronic stress, creating a self-reinforcing loop. Breaking it requires deliberate activation of the parasympathetic nervous system through consistent recovery practices—not the elimination of stress, but the restoration of recovery.
- Evidence-based sleep optimization—consistent sleep-wake schedule, strategic light management, thermal environment, addressing sleep disruptors, and evaluating for sleep apnea—produces measurable improvements in metabolic markers within weeks.
- Controlled breathing, mindfulness practice, nature exposure, and social connection all produce documented cortisol reductions and improvements in metabolic health markers. Two to five minutes of daily breathing practice is a genuine and accessible entry point.
- Thyroid dysfunction and sex hormone changes are frequently underdiagnosed contributors to metabolic dysfunction in MASLD and warrant discussion with a healthcare provider when standard lifestyle interventions produce insufficient results.

With the foundational lifestyle pillars in place—nutrition, movement, weight management, sleep, and stress—the next layer of the strategy addresses the gut. Chapter 8 explores the gut-liver axis in detail: how your microbiome either drives or defends against liver inflammation, and what targeted interventions can shift this balance in your favor.

CHAPTER 8

The Gut-Liver Axis

Healing from the Inside Out

Imagine two people following an identical diet. Same foods, same portions, same meal timing. After twelve weeks, one person shows a 35 percent reduction in liver fat. The other shows almost none.

Researchers studying dietary interventions in fatty liver disease encounter this kind of variation routinely, and for a long time it was chalked up to genetic differences or unreported dietary deviation. More recent science points to a different explanation: the microbiome.[163] The trillions of microorganisms living in the gut process food, generate metabolic byproducts, and communicate with the liver through mechanisms that are as individual as a fingerprint. Two people eating identically may be delivering very different signals to their livers—because the gut ecosystems doing the processing are nothing alike.

This is the gut-liver axis: the dynamic, bidirectional highway of communication between your intestinal microbiome and your liver. It is one of the most rapidly advancing areas of MASLD research, and it is producing some of the most actionable insights in the entire field. Understanding it helps explain why dietary improvements sometimes work faster than expected, why they sometimes work slower, and what targeted strategies can amplify the results of everything else you are doing.

Your Microbiome: A Metabolic Organ in Its Own Right

The human gut houses approximately 38 trillion microbial cells—bacteria, fungi, archaea, and viruses—collectively encoding more than 150 times the number of genes in the human genome.[164,165,166] This community, called the gut microbiome, is not a passive bystander in human metabolism. It is an active participant.

A healthy, diverse microbiome performs functions that are genuinely indispensable to metabolic health. It ferments dietary fiber that human digestive enzymes cannot break down, producing short-chain fatty acids (SCFAs)—particularly butyrate, propionate, and acetate—that serve as fuel for intestinal cells, regulate immune function, suppress inflammation, and improve insulin sensitivity throughout the body. It synthesizes certain B vitamins and vitamin K. It modulates bile acid metabolism in ways that influence both fat digestion and metabolic signaling. It regulates the expression of genes involved in fat storage and energy expenditure in the host.

When this ecosystem is diverse and balanced—well-stocked with fiber-fermenting, SCFA-producing bacteria like *Faecalibacterium prausnitzii*, *Akkermansia muciniphila*, and various *Bifidobacterium* and *Lactobacillus* species—it actively protects the liver from the inflammatory inputs that drive fatty liver disease.[167,168,169] When it is disrupted—depleted of diversity, overpopulated with harmful strains, or shifted toward fermentation pathways that produce harmful byproducts—it becomes one of the most significant sources of metabolic stress the liver faces.[170]

Dysbiosis: When the Microbiome Works Against the Liver

Dysbiosis—microbial imbalance in the gut—is consistently found in people with fatty liver disease, and the correlation strengthens with disease severity.[171] People with simple steatosis show measurable differences in microbiome composition compared to healthy controls. People with MASH show more pronounced differences. People with fibrosis and cirrhosis show the most dramatic shifts.

This is not merely correlation. Multiple lines of evidence now establish that gut dysbiosis actively contributes to fatty liver disease through specific, identifiable mechanisms—and that correcting it produces measurable improvements in liver health.

Mechanism 1: Intestinal Permeability and Endotoxin Translocation

Under healthy conditions, the intestinal lining acts as a highly selective barrier. A single layer of epithelial cells, connected by tight junction proteins, allows nutrients to pass into circulation while keeping bacteria and their byproducts contained within the gut. This barrier is not passive—it requires constant maintenance, fueled largely by butyrate produced by fiber-fermenting bacteria.

When dysbiosis depletes butyrate-producing bacteria, the tight junctions begin to loosen. The barrier becomes selectively permeable to things it should not be permeable to—including lipopolysaccharides, or LPS, a structural component of the outer membrane of gram-negative bacteria. LPS is a potent inflammatory trigger. When it crosses a compromised gut barrier and enters the portal circulation, it arrives directly at the liver, where it activates Toll-like receptor 4 (TLR4) signaling and triggers an immune response.[172]

This is not a dramatic, acute event—it is a chronic, low-level inflammatory stimulus that the liver manages around the clock in people with dysbiosis and increased intestinal permeability. The cumulative effect of this constant endotoxin exposure is sustained liver inflammation, which is the primary driver of progression from simple steatosis to MASH and fibrosis.

The popular term "leaky gut" captures this concept, though it has been so overused in wellness marketing that it deserves a more precise framing. Increased intestinal permeability is a real, measurable, clinically relevant phenomenon with specific mechanisms and documented consequences for liver health. It is not a metaphor, and it is not the explanation for every possible symptom—but in the context of fatty liver disease, it is genuinely important.

Mechanism 2: Endogenous Alcohol Production

There is one more gut-liver connection worth understanding, because it surprises nearly everyone who hears it: Some people with fatty liver disease are, in a very real sense, producing their own alcohol—without drinking a drop.

Certain bacteria and fungi that can overpopulate the gut in the context of dysbiosis are highly efficient fermenters. When fed a steady supply of simple sugars and refined carbohydrates, strains such as specific variants of *Klebsiella pneumoniae, Escherichia coli, Enterocloster bolteae*, and yeasts including *Candida* and *Pichia kudriavzevii* convert those dietary sugars into ethanol as a metabolic byproduct.[173] That ethanol does not stay in the gut. It travels directly to the liver via the portal vein—the same blood supply that carries nutrients from the digestive system—where the liver attempts to process it exactly as it would alcohol consumed in a drink.[174]

The breakdown generates acetaldehyde, a highly toxic intermediate that drives oxidative stress, damages mitochondria, triggers inflammation, and activates the scarring process in the liver.[175,176] Research published in 2022 measured ethanol concentrations in the portal blood of MASLD patients and concluded that gut-derived ethanol alone is sufficient to drive fatty liver development and progression.[177] Individuals with MASLD consistently show higher levels of these ethanol-producing microbes than healthy controls, and the correlation is strongest in people who eat high-sugar, high-fructose diets—which provides precisely the fermentation fuel these bacteria require.

In the most pronounced cases, this process produces enough ethanol to cause measurable blood alcohol levels after a carbohydrate-rich meal—a phenomenon known as auto-brewery syndrome, which is more common in people with MASLD than in the general population. The practical implication cuts in two directions: Reducing dietary sugar starves the fermentation pathway at its source, and restoring a healthier microbiome reduces the population of microbes doing the fermenting. Both strategies are within reach, and together they address what is, for some people, one of the most underappreciated drivers of liver inflammation in this disease.

Mechanism 3: Altered Short-Chain Fatty Acid Production

When the microbiome shifts away from fiber-fermenting, SCFA-producing bacteria, the consequences extend well beyond gut barrier integrity. Butyrate, propionate, and acetate produced in healthy amounts by a well-fed microbiome perform a wide range of liver-protective functions: They reduce hepatic fat accumulation, improve insulin sensitivity, lower inflammatory cytokine production, and support the integrity of the gut barrier that protects the liver from endotoxin exposure.[178]

In people with dysbiosis—particularly those eating low-fiber, high-sugar diets—SCFA production declines significantly. The liver loses these protective signals. And without the butyrate that fuels intestinal cells, the gut barrier weakens further, increasing endotoxin translocation in a self-reinforcing cycle: Less fiber leads to less butyrate, less butyrate weakens the barrier, a weakened barrier exposes the liver to more LPS, more LPS drives liver inflammation, and liver inflammation worsens the metabolic environment that sustains dysbiosis. It's like a building where the power grid fails, the security doors unlock, and an arsonist walks in—each failure not only causes damage but ensures the next one is more destructive.

Increasing dietary fiber is the most direct intervention for restoring SCFA production—and among the most impactful gut-health strategies available.

Food Diversity: The Most Underrated Microbiome Strategy

The single most important predictor of a healthy, resilient microbiome is dietary diversity—the number of different plant foods (grains, veggies, fruits, legumes, nuts, seeds, herbs, and spices) consumed on a regular basis. This finding emerges consistently across the largest microbiome research projects, including the American Gut Project, which analyzed microbiome samples from thousands of participants across multiple countries.[179]

People who eat 30 or more different plant foods per week show significantly greater microbiome diversity, higher populations of beneficial bacteria, and more robust SCFA production than those eating fewer than ten different plant foods per week. The difference is not subtle—it is among the strongest dietary predictors of microbiome health identified in population-scale research.

This framing—counting diversity rather than restricting categories—is both more accurate and more sustainable than elimination-based dietary advice. It shifts the focus from what to remove to what to add. Every new plant food, herb, spice, bean, or grain introduces fiber types and polyphenols that feed slightly different microbial populations, gradually expanding the diversity and functional resilience of the ecosystem.

Thirty different plants per week sounds ambitious until you start counting. A single meal of a mixed salad with five vegetables, dressed with olive oil and sprinkled with sesame seeds, represents seven to eight plants. A smoothie with spinach, frozen berries, banana, and flaxseed adds four more. Herbs and spices count—a meal seasoned with garlic, cumin, and turmeric adds three. The target is achievable with intention, and the microbiome benefits accumulate over weeks.

Fiber: The Foundation of Gut-Liver Health

Dietary fiber is the primary fuel of a healthy microbiome—and the single most consistently evidence-supported dietary intervention for gut health in the context of fatty liver disease. It is not glamorous, it does not come in a capsule, and it does not carry the excitement of emerging therapies.[180] It works, reliably, at scale, in virtually every study that has examined it.

Not all fiber is metabolically equivalent, however. The research increasingly distinguishes between fiber types based on their fermentability, their specific effects on microbial populations, and their impact on SCFA production and liver health.

- **Soluble fiber (oats, legumes, apples, psyllium, flaxseed):** Dissolves in water to form a gel that slows glucose absorption, moderates insulin response, feeds *Bifidobacterium* and other beneficial bacteria, and generates butyrate and propionate.[181] Consistently associated with improvements in liver enzymes and metabolic markers in clinical trials.[182]
- **Insoluble fiber (whole grains, vegetables, wheat bran):** Does not dissolve but adds bulk, accelerates gut transit, and reduces exposure time of the gut lining to potentially harmful substances. Supports regular bowel habits and reduces intestinal permeability indirectly by keeping gut contents moving.
- **Resistant starch (found in cooked-and-cooled potatoes and rice, raw green bananas, legumes, oats):** Passes through the small intestine undigested and is fermented in the colon, producing particularly robust butyrate generation.[183] One randomized controlled trial found that resistant starch supplementation reduced intrahepatic triglycerides by approximately eight percent through microbiome modulation—a meaningful effect delivered through dietary modification alone.[184] Essentially, resistant starch "scrubs" the fat out of your liver.
- **Prebiotic fiber (inulin, fructooligosaccharides, galacto-oligosaccharides—found in garlic, onions, leeks, asparagus, bananas, chicory):** Selectively promotes the growth of *Bifidobacterium* and *Akkermansia*

muciniphila—species particularly associated with improved gut barrier function, lower systemic inflammation, and better insulin sensitivity.[185] These are among the most targeted fiber types for microbiome support.

The practical target for adults is a minimum of 25 to 35 grams of fiber per day from whole food sources. Most people eating a typical Western diet consume approximately 12 to 15 grams. The gap between current intake and a therapeutic target is significant—and the most effective way to close it is not a fiber supplement but a gradual, sustained increase in vegetables, legumes, whole grains, nuts, seeds, and fruit. If you struggle to get the recommended fiber from dietary sources alone, a high-quality fiber supplement can be helpful.

One important note on the pace of fiber increase: The gut microbiome adapts to dietary changes, but it does so over days to weeks. Rapidly increasing fiber intake from a low baseline commonly produces bloating, gas, and digestive discomfort as the microbial population adjusts. Increasing fiber gradually—adding one or two servings of high-fiber foods per week rather than overhauling the diet overnight—allows the microbiome to adapt with minimal discomfort.

Fermented Foods: Live Cultures from the Table, Not the Bottle

Fermented foods—those produced through the controlled activity of microorganisms—have been part of human diets for thousands of years. Only recently has research begun to quantify what traditional food cultures appear to have understood intuitively: Regular consumption of fermented foods measurably improves microbiome diversity and reduces markers of systemic inflammation.

A landmark 2021 randomized controlled trial from Stanford University compared the effects of a high-fiber diet to a high-fermented-food diet over ten weeks.[186] While both groups showed metabolic improvements, the fermented food group showed greater increases in microbiome diversity—one of the most important metrics of gut health—and greater reductions in 19 inflammatory proteins, including cytokines directly implicated in fatty liver disease.

The most accessible and well-studied fermented foods for regular consumption include plain yogurt, kefir, sauerkraut, kimchi, tempeh, miso, and kombucha. Each delivers live bacterial cultures with slightly different microbial profiles, making variety across fermented foods more beneficial than relying exclusively on one.

- **Plain yogurt and kefir:** Among the most practical and widely available sources of live cultures. Kefir typically contains a broader range of bacterial and yeast species than yogurt and is well-tolerated even by many people with lactose sensitivity, as the fermentation process substantially reduces lactose content.[187] the fermentation process actually "pre-digests" the milk for you. The healthy bacteria in kefir grains eat up the lactose (milk sugar) and turn it into lactic acid. By the time you drink it, the lactose is significantly reduced and the kefir is packed with the very enzymes your body needs to digest it smoothly. It's a way to get the benefits of dairy and probiotics without the digestive distress. Choose products with live and active cultures and without added sugars.
- **Sauerkraut and kimchi:** Fermented cabbage preparations that are rich in *Lactobacillus* species. The key is choosing unpasteurized versions—heat processing kills the

live cultures that provide the microbiome benefit. Look for products sold refrigerated, not shelf-stable.

- **Tempeh:** A fermented soy product with a denser nutrient profile than tofu, delivering both protein and probiotic benefit. It is also a meaningful source of plant-based protein for those reducing meat intake.
- **Miso:** A fermented soybean paste used in soups and sauces. Rich in live cultures and also a source of prebiotic compounds. Opt for traditional, unpasteurized varieties where available.
- **Kombucha:** A fermented tea with a growing evidence base for microbiome benefit, though the variety of bacterial strains and their concentrations varies considerably between products. Choose low-sugar varieties—some commercial kombuchas contain nearly as much sugar as a soft drink, which undermines the benefit.

Probiotics and Synbiotics: When Supplements Add Value

The supplement industry has enthusiastically embraced probiotics, producing a market so crowded and inconsistently standardized that it is difficult for most people to identify what actually works. The evidence is more nuanced than either probiotic advocates or skeptics tend to acknowledge.

For fatty liver disease specifically, the research on probiotic supplementation is genuinely encouraging. Multiple meta-analyses of randomized controlled trials have found that multi-strain probiotic supplementation—particularly combinations of *Lactobacillus* and *Bifidobacterium* species—produces consistent, modest improvements in liver enzymes (ALT and AST), reduction in liver fat, improvements in insulin resistance markers, and reductions in inflammatory cytokines when used for eight to twelve weeks or longer.[188]

Taking a high-quality, multi-strain probiotic is like sending a specialized repair crew into your digestive system. Research shows that after about two or three months, these beneficial bacteria can significantly lower your liver enzymes and reduce liver fat. They do this by fixing your gut lining—preventing toxins from leaking into your bloodstream and attacking your liver. It's not a quick fix, but it's a powerful way to calm down the inflammation in your body and help your liver metabolism get back on track.

The keyword is multi-strain. Single-strain probiotics show less consistent benefit than combinations, which more closely approximate the complexity of a healthy microbiome. The strains with the most evidence for MASLD include *Lactobacillus rhamnosus, Lactobacillus acidophilus, Lactobacillus casei, Bifidobacterium longum*, and *Bifidobacterium breve*—not all of which are present in every commercial product.[189]

Synbiotics—combinations of probiotics and prebiotics designed to improve the survival and implantation of the live cultures—show additive benefit over either alone in several trials. The prebiotic component provides the fermentation substrate the probiotic bacteria need to establish themselves and thrive, rather than simply passing through the gut without taking hold.

> **How to Choose a Probiotic Worth Taking.** *Look for products that specify strains by full name (genus, species, and strain designation—not just "Lactobacillus acidophilus" but "Lactobacillus acidophilus NCFM," for example). Viable cell count at expiration rather than at*

> *manufacture matters—look for products that guarantee potency through the best-by date. Choose products requiring refrigeration or specifically engineered for shelf stability. Multi-strain formulations of five or more strains with a combined count of 10 to 50 billion CFU are the products most studied in MASLD trials. And pair your probiotic with increased prebiotic fiber from food—a probiotic taken alongside a low-fiber diet is working at a significant disadvantage.*

Targeting Harmful Microbes: The Role of Diet and Selective Intervention

Given what we now know about ethanol-producing bacteria in the gut and their contribution to liver inflammation, a logical question arises: Can we do something specifically to reduce these harmful populations, rather than just generally supporting beneficial ones?

The answer is yes—and the most powerful tool available is also the most fundamental: reducing dietary sugar and refined carbohydrates.

The ethanol-producing strains—*Klebsiella pneumoniae*, certain *E. coli* variants, *Candida* and related yeasts—are overwhelmingly dependent on a high-sugar, high-fructose fermentation fuels. Remove the fuel and you remove the competitive advantage of these organisms. A Mediterranean-style or lower-carbohydrate dietary pattern consistently shifts the microbiome away from these harmful fermenters and toward fiber-dependent, SCFA-producing species—not because it directly targets the bacteria, but because it changes the nutritional environment they compete in.

Polyphenol-rich foods add another layer of targeted antimicrobial activity. Compounds found in berries, olive oil, green tea, dark chocolate, garlic, and oregano have demonstrated selective inhibitory activity against microbiome-disrupting gram-negative bacteria and *Candida* species in multiple research settings—while largely sparing or supporting beneficial bacterial populations. This selectivity is a meaningful advantage over broad-spectrum interventions. The garlic on your roasted vegetables and the olive oil in your salad dressing are, among other things, gently modulating the microbial environment of your gut.

For people with significant gut dysbiosis or suspected small intestinal bacterial overgrowth (SIBO)—characterized by chronic bloating, gas, irregular bowel habits, and abdominal distension, particularly after carbohydrate-rich meals—evaluation by a gastroenterologist is warranted. Specific breath testing can identify SIBO, and treatment protocols exist that go beyond dietary modification. This is an area where a knowledgeable clinician can be genuinely helpful, particularly when standard dietary improvements produce limited gut symptom relief.

Fecal Microbiota Transplantation: The Most Powerful Reset Available

Fecal microbiota transplantation (FMT)—the transfer of processed stool from a carefully screened healthy donor into the gut of a patient—is the most direct and comprehensive method available for resetting a severely dysbiotic gut microbiome. It is not a fringe therapy. It is an FDA-approved treatment for recurrent *Clostridioides difficile* infection, with cure rates exceeding 90 percent, and it is under active investigation for MASLD, inflammatory bowel disease, and metabolic syndrome.

In early trials of FMT for MASLD, transplantation from metabolically healthy lean donors has shown promising results: improvements in insulin sensitivity, reductions in liver fat, measurable shifts in microbiome composition toward healthier profiles, and reductions in ethanol-producing bacterial strains.[190] The effects are, in some cases, more rapid and pronounced than those achieved through dietary intervention alone—which makes biological sense, given that FMT directly displaces the harmful microbial populations rather than simply creating conditions less favorable to them.

FMT for MASLD is not yet standard care. The trials to date have been small, the protocols are not standardized, and the long-term durability of microbiome changes from FMT—particularly without sustained dietary support—is not fully established. The effects appear to be donor-dependent, meaning outcomes vary based on the microbial profile of the specific donor used.

For most people reading this book, FMT is not a near-term option. It is worth knowing about as an emerging therapy that may become more accessible and more standardized over the coming years—particularly for people with advanced disease or severely dysbiotic gut profiles that have not responded to dietary and probiotic intervention. If you are working with a hepatologist or gastroenterologist, it is a reasonable topic to raise in the context of a comprehensive management discussion.

Emerging Microbiome Therapies: What Is Coming

The microbiome field is advancing rapidly, and several therapeutic approaches currently in development are likely to become clinically meaningful in the next five to ten years.

- **Postbiotics:** Rather than delivering live bacteria (probiotics) or food for those bacteria (prebiotics), postbiotics are the bioactive compounds produced by bacteria—things like butyrate itself, specific peptides, or inactivated microbial cell walls. Postbiotics bypass the variability of live culture supplementation and deliver the beneficial compounds directly. Early research shows anti-inflammatory and gut-barrier-supportive effects.[191] Butyrate supplementation in particular has shown promising effects on liver inflammation in preliminary nonhuman trials.[192]

- **Bacteriophage therapy:** Bacteriophages, or phages for short, are viruses that selectively infect and kill specific bacterial strains without disturbing the broader microbial ecosystem. Preclinical research has demonstrated that phages targeting high-alcohol-producing *Klebsiella pneumoniae* strains reduce ethanol production and liver fat accumulation in animal models.[193] Additionally, small clinical trials, case reports, and animal models document phage therapy effectiveness against *E. coli, A. baumannii, and E. faecalis*, highlighting phage therapy as a targeted approach to liver diseases.[194] This represents one of the most mechanistically precise approaches to microbiome intervention for MASLD currently under investigation.

- **Precision microbiome modulation:** Microbiome testing is advancing toward a level of specificity where individual dysbiosis profiles can be mapped and targeted interventions—specific probiotic strains, prebiotic types, or phage combinations—can be tailored to the individual's baseline composition. Early research on personalized nutrition based on microbiome profiling has produced significantly better metabolic outcomes than generalized dietary advice.[195] This approach is not yet widely accessible but is moving toward clinical utility.

- **Next-generation probiotics:** Engineered or selectively cultured bacterial strains with enhanced therapeutic properties—such as acetaldehyde-degrading *Lactobacillus* strains designed specifically to counteract endogenous alcohol production—are in development and early-phase clinical trials. These represent a more targeted evolution beyond the generalist multi-strain products currently available.

The Practical Hierarchy: Where to Start and How to Build

Given the range of gut health interventions available—from food diversity to fiber to fermented foods to probiotics to emerging therapies—it helps to have a clear prioritization framework. The following hierarchy reflects the evidence base and practical accessibility of each layer.

Foundation — Dietary optimization: Reduce sugar and refined carbohydrates (removes fermentation fuel for harmful bacteria), increase plant food diversity toward 30 or more types per week, and increase total fiber intake toward 30 grams per day from whole food sources. This single layer addresses the gut microbiome more comprehensively than any supplement protocol stacked on top of a poor diet.

Layer 2 — Targeted fiber and resistant starch: Deliberately include resistant starch sources (cooled cooked potatoes or rice, green bananas, legumes) and prebiotic-rich foods (garlic, onions, leeks, asparagus, oats) to selectively support the most beneficial microbial populations. These can be added to an already improving diet for amplified effect.

Layer 3 — Fermented foods: Add one to two servings of fermented foods daily—plain yogurt, kefir, sauerkraut, kimchi, or tempeh. Consistent daily consumption, rather than occasional large amounts, produces the most meaningful microbiome shifts.

Layer 4 — Probiotic supplementation: A high-quality, multi-strain probiotic is one of the most broadly beneficial supplements most people can take—not a targeted intervention for specific symptoms, but a foundational support for overall health. The modern diet, repeated antibiotic exposure, chronic stress, and disrupted sleep all degrade the microbiome steadily over time, and most people are not replacing what is lost through food alone. For people with fatty liver disease specifically, the documented improvements in liver enzymes, liver fat, and insulin resistance markers seen in clinical trials make daily probiotic use a logical and low-risk addition to any management protocol. Use a multi-strain product with at least five to ten strains and a guaranteed potency of 10 to 50 billion CFU through the expiration date—not just at manufacture. Pair it with increased dietary fiber, which provides the fermentation substrate the probiotic bacteria need to survive and establish themselves. Plan on a minimum of eight to twelve weeks of consistent use before assessing benefit, and treat it as an ongoing daily habit rather than a short-term course.

Layer 5 — Advanced interventions: For people with persistent, significant gut dysfunction despite dietary and probiotic intervention, consultation with a gastroenterologist for SIBO testing, microbiome analysis, or discussion of FMT is appropriate. These are not first-line strategies but have genuine utility for the subset of people who need them.

Start Here: Your Gut Health Reset Protocol

Week 1 – Remove the Fuel

- Eliminate or dramatically reduce sugar-sweetened beverages and high-fructose corn syrup products—this single change begins to starve the ethanol-producing bacteria within days
- Replace at least one refined carbohydrate per day with a whole food alternative: white rice with legumes, crackers with vegetable sticks, sweetened yogurt with plain yogurt
- Count the number of different plant foods you ate this week—most people discover the number is lower than they expect

Week 2 – Feed the Beneficial Bacteria

- Add one new plant food to your diet that you do not currently eat regularly—a new legume, vegetable, nut, or grain
- Include at least one prebiotic-rich food daily: garlic, onions, leeks, asparagus, oats, or green bananas
- Begin increasing total fiber intake gradually—add one high-fiber food per day and observe how your digestive system responds

Week 3 – Introduce Live Cultures

- Add one serving of a fermented food daily—plain yogurt, kefir, or a small portion of sauerkraut or kimchi

- If starting a probiotic supplement, begin now—alongside the dietary fiber improvements already in place
- Note any changes in digestive symptoms: Bloating, regularity, and discomfort are practical early indicators that the microbiome is responding

Ongoing – Sustain and Diversify

- Track your weekly plant food diversity—aim to increase the number of different plants by two to three per week until you consistently reach 25 to 30
- Rotate your fermented food sources—vary between yogurt, kefir, kimchi, sauerkraut, and tempeh to introduce different microbial profiles
- Consider a microbiome stool test if available and accessible—several direct-to-consumer options provide useful baseline data, though interpretation should be approached with appropriate skepticism given the still-developing state of this science

> ***The Gut-Liver Connection in Practice.*** *Every dietary improvement you make for your liver is simultaneously an improvement for your gut microbiome—and vice versa. Reducing sugar, increasing fiber, eating more polyphenol-rich plants, improving sleep, and managing stress all shift the microbial environment toward less fermentation of harmful byproducts, better short-chain fatty acid production, and a stronger gut barrier. The gut-liver axis is not a separate intervention—it is the same intervention, viewed from a different angle.*

Key Takeaways

- The gut microbiome is a metabolic organ that either actively protects or actively harms the liver, depending on its composition. Dysbiosis—microbial imbalance—is consistently found in people with fatty liver disease and worsens with disease severity.
- Increased intestinal permeability allows bacterial endotoxins (LPS) to enter the portal circulation and trigger chronic liver inflammation. This is driven by depletion of butyrate-producing bacteria and is directly addressable through dietary fiber.
- Certain dysbiotic bacteria and yeasts produce ethanol from dietary sugars through fermentation, exposing the liver to a constant trickle of alcohol-like toxins even in nondrinkers. Reducing dietary sugar removes the fermentation fuel; restoring microbiome diversity reduces the population of microbes producing it.
- Dietary diversity—targeting 30 or more different plant foods per week—is the most powerful predictor of a healthy, resilient microbiome. Fiber quantity and variety (including resistant starch and prebiotic fiber types) directly supports SCFA production and gut barrier integrity.
- Fermented foods consumed daily produce measurable improvements in microbiome diversity and reductions in inflammatory markers. Unpasteurized, refrigerated products deliver live cultures; variety across fermented food types introduces different beneficial microbial profiles.

- Multi-strain probiotic supplementation produces consistent modest improvements in liver enzymes, liver fat, and insulin resistance markers in clinical trials when used for eight to twelve weeks alongside dietary fiber. Strain specificity and quality matter—not all probiotics are equivalent.
- The hierarchy of gut health intervention runs from dietary foundation (reduce sugar, increase fiber and plant diversity) through fermented foods and targeted probiotics to advanced interventions like FMT for appropriate candidates. Supplements layer on top of—never replace—dietary improvement.

With the gut-liver axis addressed, the next chapter turns to the supplements with the strongest evidence for directly supporting liver repair and metabolic health. Chapter 9 provides a rigorous, balanced assessment of what the research actually shows—and what it doesn't—so you can make informed decisions about which supplements genuinely deserve a place in your protocol.

CHAPTER 9

Evidence-Based Supplements

What the Research Actually Shows

The supplement aisle is a confident place. Every bottle promises something. Detox. Liver cleanse. Metabolic support. Fat burner. The labels are bold, the claims are sweeping, and the price points range from modest to genuinely surprising. And if you have spent any time recently searching for information about liver health or metabolic disease, targeted social media advertising has almost certainly ensured that a new supplement designed specifically for your needs appears in your feed on a near-weekly basis—each one positioned as the missing piece you have not yet tried. For someone diagnosed with fatty liver disease and motivated to do something about it, this combination of shelf and screen can feel like either an opportunity or an overwhelming maze.

The honest answer is that they are neither, exactly. Some supplements have a meaningful, evidence-supported role in a comprehensive MASLD management strategy. Others have preliminary promise but insufficient human data to justify confident recommendations. And many—including the majority of products marketed specifically as "liver cleanses" or "detox" formulas—have little to no rigorous evidence behind them.

This chapter cuts through that noise with a rigorous but accessible assessment of what the research actually shows. The goal is not to build the longest possible supplement protocol—adding a dozen capsules to a day while the foundational lifestyle work remains undone is an expensive way to achieve minimal results. The goal is to identify the specific supplements for which the evidence is genuinely compelling, understand the mechanisms by which they work, know who is most likely to benefit, and use them intelligently as a layer of support on top of—never instead of—the dietary, exercise, sleep, and gut health foundations established in previous chapters.

> **The Non-Negotiable Principle of This Chapter.** *Supplements support lifestyle—they do not replace it. The most impressive supplement protocol built on a foundation of poor diet, inactivity, inadequate sleep, and chronic stress will produce a fraction of the benefit achievable through lifestyle alone. Every supplement discussed in this chapter works best when the lifestyle conditions that make it possible are already in place.*

Tier 1: Strongest Evidence for MASLD

The following supplements have the most consistent, most replicated evidence base for meaningful benefit in fatty liver disease and its metabolic drivers. They have plausible mechanisms, human clinical trial data, and reasonable safety profiles at therapeutic doses.

Omega-3 Fatty Acids (EPA and DHA)

Omega-3 fatty acids—specifically eicosapentaenoic acid (EPA) and docosahexaenoic acid (DHA), found in fatty fish and fish oil supplements—have some of the strongest and most consistent evidence bases of any supplement studied in MASLD.

The mechanisms are well-characterized. EPA and DHA activate PPAR-alpha, a nuclear receptor that upregulates the liver's fat-burning pathways and suppresses *de novo* lipogenesis—the process by which the liver manufactures new fat from carbohydrates.[196] They also reduce the liver's production of triglycerides, lower systemic inflammation through conversion to anti-inflammatory prostaglandins and resolvins, and improve insulin sensitivity in liver and muscle tissue. In the gut, omega-3s support microbiome diversity and reduce intestinal permeability.[197]

Multiple meta-analyses of randomized controlled trials have found that omega-3 supplementation significantly reduces liver fat, lowers ALT and AST levels, reduces liver stiffness in early fibrosis, and improves triglycerides and HDL cholesterol in people with MASLD.[198,199,200] The most consistent benefits appear at doses of 2 to 4 grams of combined EPA and DHA per day—considerably more than the 300-miligram doses found in many standard fish oil capsules.

Dietary sources remain the gold standard: Two to three servings of fatty fish per week (salmon, sardines, mackerel, anchovies) deliver meaningful EPA and DHA alongside protein and other liver-supportive nutrients. For those who do not eat fatty fish regularly, a high-quality concentrated fish oil or algae-derived omega-3 supplement (the latter suitable for vegetarians and vegans) at 2 to 4 grams combined EPA/DHA daily is a well-supported addition to a liver health protocol.

Quality matters considerably in omega-3 supplements. Fish oil oxidizes readily, and rancid fish oil may deliver more harm than benefit. Choose products from reputable manufacturers that provide third-party testing for purity and oxidation levels (peroxide value and

TOTOX score). Enteric-coated capsules reduce fishy aftertaste and improve tolerance. Algae-based omega-3s avoid the oxidation concerns of fish-derived products and are equally bioavailable. Re-esterified triglyceride (rTG) fish oil is more easily absorbed by the body compared to other forms like ethyl esters (EE), leading to more effective utilization of the beneficial fatty acids.

One of the most actionable advances in omega-3 supplementation is the availability of a simple blood test—the omega-3 index—that measures the actual percentage of EPA and DHA in red blood cell membranes. Unlike a dietary recall or a supplement label, this test tells you what your tissues actually contain. An omega-3 index below 4% is associated with increased cardiovascular risk and poor inflammatory control. An index of 8–12% is the evidence-based optimal range and is associated with meaningful reductions in liver fat accumulation, lower pro-inflammatory cytokines (IL-6 and TNF-alpha), reduced ALT and AST levels, and emerging evidence suggesting a slowing of fibrosis progression. Many people supplementing with standard-dose fish oil remain in the 4–6% range—enough to see some benefit, but not enough to reach the therapeutic threshold where the most significant liver and metabolic effects are documented. If you are taking omega-3s for liver health, testing your omega-3 index at baseline and after three to four months of supplementation is the most direct way to confirm your dose is actually working. Home finger-prick tests are now widely available and reasonably priced.

Vitamin E

Vitamin E—specifically the alpha-tocopherol form—is one of the few supplements to have been studied in a rigorous, large-scale clinical trial specifically for MASH (the more advanced, inflammatory form of fatty liver disease). The PIVENS trial, published in the *New England Journal of Medicine*, found that 800 IU per day of vitamin E produced significant histological improvement in nondiabetic adults with MASH—including reductions in liver fat, inflammation, and ballooning degeneration of liver cells.[201]

The mechanism is primarily antioxidant. MASH is driven in part by oxidative stress—an excess of reactive oxygen species that damage liver cell membranes, mitochondria, and DNA. Vitamin E, as a fat-soluble antioxidant, is specifically positioned in cell membranes where oxidative damage is most concentrated, and it neutralizes these reactive species before they can trigger the inflammatory cascade.

Vitamin E is not appropriate for everyone with fatty liver disease. Current evidence supports its use most clearly in nondiabetic adults with biopsy-confirmed MASH—a more specific and advanced presentation than simple steatosis. In people with diabetes, the benefit-risk calculation is less clear, as some data suggests potential interactions with glycemic management. High-dose vitamin E (above 400 IU per day long-term) has also been associated in some analyses with a modest increase in all-cause mortality and, in men, an increased risk of prostate cancer—findings that continue to be debated but warrant caution with unsupervised high-dose supplementation.[202,203]

The practical guidance: Vitamin E at therapeutic doses for MASH is a conversation to have with the physician managing your liver care, not a self-directed decision. For people with confirmed MASH who are nondiabetic, the evidence is genuinely compelling. For those with simple steatosis, the benefit-risk calculation is less clear-cut.

Vitamin B3 (Niacin and Niacinamide)

Vitamin B3 has emerged as a particularly interesting supplement in the MASLD landscape through a recently elucidated mechanism that connects it directly to the genetic drivers of fatty liver disease.

Research published in the journal *Metabolism* in 2025 identified that hepatic microRNA-93—a small regulatory RNA molecule—promotes the development and progression of MASLD by suppressing SIRT1,[204] a critical protein that governs mitochondrial function, fat oxidation, and cellular energy metabolism in the liver. Vitamin B3, in both its niacin and niacinamide forms, has been shown to effectively suppress microRNA-93 activity, thereby restoring SIRT1 function and improving the liver's capacity to metabolize fat rather than store it.

Beyond this genetic mechanism, niacin at higher doses has long been established as one of the most effective agents for raising HDL cholesterol and reducing triglycerides—two of the most important lipid parameters in MASLD management.[205] Niacinamide, the nonflushing form of B3, avoids the prostaglandin-mediated flushing response that makes high-dose niacin uncomfortable for many people while retaining meaningful metabolic benefits. Niacin flushing is a temporary reaction that occurs when taking high doses of niacin, causing redness, warmth, and a tingling sensation in the skin, especially on the face and upper body. This harmless side effect usually lasts for about one to two hours and is due to the widening of blood vessels.

B3 from food sources—found in poultry, fish, legumes, whole grains, and mushrooms—supports baseline needs. Therapeutic supplementation, particularly for the microRNA-93 pathway, typically involves doses above what diet alone provides; however, high-dose niacin supplementation carries real risks including liver toxicity at very high doses (1,000 to 3,0000 mg/day), blood sugar elevation, and significant flushing. This is not a supplement to dose aggressively without medical guidance. Niacinamide at moderate doses (250 to 500 mg per day) carries a considerably more favorable safety profile and is the more appropriate form for unsupervised use.

Berberine

Berberine is an alkaloid compound found in several plants, including barberry (*Berberis vulgaris*), goldenseal (*Hydrastis canadensis*), and tree turmeric (*Berberis aristata*), and it has one of the most impressive evidence bases of any natural compound studied for metabolic health. Multiple meta-analyses show that berberine at typical doses of 900 to 1,500 mg per day (divided into two or three doses with meals) consistently reduces fasting glucose, HbA1c, fasting insulin, and the HOMA-IR measure of insulin resistance in people with type 2 diabetes, prediabetes, metabolic syndrome, and MASLD.[206,207,208] The glycemic effects are comparable to metformin in head-to-head trials—a comparison that gets berberine considerable attention in integrative medicine circles.[209]

The primary mechanism is AMPK activation. AMPK (adenosine monophosphate-activated protein kinase) is often described as the cell's master metabolic switch—it is activated by energy deficit and responds by increasing fat oxidation, improving insulin sensitivity, reducing hepatic glucose production, and suppressing *de novo* lipogenesis. This is the same pathway activated by exercise and metformin, which explains why berberine's metabolic effects resemble both.

Berberine also beneficially modulates the gut microbiome—increasing *Akkermansia muciniphila* and other SCFA-producing species, reducing ethanol-producing gram-negative bacteria, and improving gut barrier integrity.[210] It has additional effects on lipid metabolism, reducing triglycerides and LDL cholesterol in most trials. For people with MASLD complicated by insulin resistance, prediabetes, or dyslipidemia—which describes a significant proportion of those with the condition—berberine addresses multiple root causes simultaneously.

Safety is generally favorable at standard doses, though berberine should not be combined with metformin without medical supervision due to potential additive effects on blood sugar. It can interact with cytochrome P450 enzymes and may affect the metabolism of some medications. Gastrointestinal side effects—bloating, constipation, or loose stools—are the most common adverse effects and are usually dose-dependent and manageable by starting at a lower dose and titrating up. Pregnant or breastfeeding women should avoid berberine.

Vitamin D

Vitamin D deficiency is remarkably prevalent in people with fatty liver disease—and the relationship appears to be more than incidental.[211] Recent research found that adults with vitamin D levels at or above 44 ng/mL had approximately 60 percent lower odds of having MASLD compared to those with deficient levels at or below 22 ng/mL.[212] This dose-response relationship—more vitamin D associated with meaningfully lower MASLD risk—is consistent with a causal role for vitamin D insufficiency in disease development and progression.

The mechanisms are multiple. Vitamin D receptors are expressed extensively in liver tissue, and vitamin D signaling regulates liver fat metabolism, insulin sensitivity, and the inflammatory pathways most active in MASH. Vitamin D also modulates immune function in ways that reduce the TLR4-mediated inflammatory response to bacterial endotoxins—the same endotoxin pathway that drives liver inflammation via the gut-liver axis.

Testing vitamin D status before supplementing is strongly advisable. Optimal levels for liver health appear to be at the higher end of the normal range—above 40 ng/mL (100 nmol/L)—rather than merely avoiding frank deficiency. For most people with levels below this threshold, supplemental doses of 5,000 to 10,000 IU per day of vitamin D3 (cholecalciferol, the most bioavailable form) are typically required to reach optimal levels, though individual response varies considerably. Retesting after three months of supplementation allows dose adjustment. Vitamin D3 is best absorbed when taken with a meal containing fat.

A note on vitamin D toxicity: Unlike most water-soluble vitamins, vitamin D is fat-soluble and can accumulate. True toxicity is rare and typically requires extremely high supplemental doses sustained over long periods, but it is a reason to test rather than arbitrarily supplement at very high doses.

Inositol

Inositol—particularly myo-inositol and its partner D-chiro-inositol—is a naturally occurring sugar alcohol that functions as a critical second messenger in the insulin signaling cascade. When insulin binds to its receptor on a cell surface, inositol-containing phospholipids mediate the downstream signal that tells the cell to take up glucose. For your body to use sugar for energy, a complex "relay race" has to happen inside your cells. Insulin starts the race by knocking on the cell's door, but it's a special group of molecules called inositols that actually carry the message to the rest of the cell. Think of them as the internal wiring of your metabolism. If that wiring is healthy, your cells open up and let sugar in. If the wiring is damaged—which often happens in fatty liver disease—your cells become "deaf" to insulin, and sugar builds up in your blood instead of being used for fuel. In insulin-resistant states, this signaling pathway is impaired, and inositol availability is a limiting factor in its restoration.

Meta-analyses of randomized controlled trials show that myo-inositol supplementation produces robust improvements in insulin sensitivity—standardized mean differences of 0.7 to 0.9 in HOMA-IR, a clinically meaningful effect—particularly in polyendocrine metabolic ovarian syndrome (PMOS); formerly polycystic ovary syndrome (PCOS), a condition closely associated with insulin resistance and elevated MASLD risk.[213,214] Benefits extend to general insulin resistance, prediabetes, and metabolic syndrome beyond PMOS.

The most effective approach appears to be a combination of myo-inositol and D-chiro-inositol at a 40:1 ratio, which mirrors the physiological ratio found in human plasma and tissue.[215] This combination enhances both the initial insulin receptor signaling step (myo-inositol's primary role) and the downstream glucose disposal step (D-chiro-inositol's primary role). Typical effective doses are 2 to 4 grams of myo-inositol per day combined with proportional D-chiro-inositol, taken in divided doses.

Inositol has a notably favorable safety profile—it is found naturally in many foods (citrus fruits, legumes, whole grains, and nuts) and even at supplemental doses produces minimal adverse effects beyond occasional mild gastrointestinal symptoms at higher doses. It is one of the most accessible and well-tolerated metabolic supplements available.

Chromium

Chromium is an essential trace mineral that enhances insulin action by facilitating the binding of insulin to its receptor and improving post-receptor signaling.[216] It is the oldest nutritional supplement studied for insulin resistance, and while the evidence is less dramatic than for berberine or inositol, it is consistent enough to merit inclusion in a comprehensive metabolic support protocol.

Meta-analyses of randomized controlled trials find that chromium supplementation at 200 to 1,000 micrograms per day (typically as chromium picolinate, the most bioavailable form) produces consistent reductions in fasting insulin and HOMA-IR in people with diabetes or insulin resistance.[217,218] Effects on fasting blood glucose are modest, and effects on HbA1c are variable across populations. Chromium appears to work best as an adjunct to other interventions rather than as a primary insulin-sensitizing strategy.

The most useful context for chromium supplementation is as a complement to berberine or inositol in people with significant insulin resistance—not as a first-line standalone agent. It is inexpensive, well-tolerated at standard doses, and adds a distinct mechanism to a multi-faceted metabolic support protocol. Doses above 1,000 micrograms per day are not supported by additional evidence and are not recommended.

Magnesium

Magnesium is the most overlooked mineral in metabolic health—and one of the most consequential. It is a required cofactor in more than 300 enzymatic reactions in the human body, including the activation of the insulin receptor itself.[219] Without adequate intracellular magnesium, the molecular machinery that allows cells to respond to insulin cannot function properly—making magnesium deficiency a direct, mechanistic contributor to insulin resistance, and therefore to fatty liver disease.

The problem is both common and routinely missed. An estimated 50 to 80 percent of people with metabolic syndrome have suboptimal magnesium status—yet standard serum magnesium tests almost never detect it.[220] Because over 99 percent of the body's magnesium is stored inside cells and bone, serum levels remain in the normal range until deficiency is severe. RBC (red blood cell) magnesium is the appropriate functional test for anyone who wants to actually assess their status.

The clinical evidence for magnesium supplementation in insulin resistance is consistent: Multiple meta-analyses of randomized controlled trials find meaningful reductions in fasting insulin, fasting glucose, and HOMA-IR in magnesium-deficient adults who supplement—with benefits most pronounced in people with insulin resistance, prediabetes, and type 2 diabetes.[221,222] Magnesium also reduces hsCRP and IL-6, two of the inflammatory markers most directly implicated in MASH progression, and it improves sleep quality through GABA receptor activation and nocturnal cortisol reduction—addressing the sleep-insulin resistance pathway discussed in Chapter 7 through a direct nutritional mechanism.[223]

Form matters considerably. Magnesium glycinate and magnesium malate are the most bioavailable forms for systemic metabolic effects and are the best tolerated—magnesium oxide, the most common and cheapest form found in standard multivitamins, is poorly absorbed and essentially useless for correcting deficiency. Standard therapeutic doses are 300 to 400 mg of elemental magnesium daily in divided doses, typically with meals. Loose stools are the dose-limiting side effect and can guide individual titration (gradually adjusting dose to find your optimal amount)—if this occurs, reduce the dose and increase gradually.

Given its prevalence of deficiency in the target population, its direct mechanistic role in insulin signaling, and its exceptional safety and cost profile, magnesium is one of the most justifiable first supplements to address—ideally after confirming status with RBC magnesium testing, and before adding more complex or expensive interventions.

Choline

Choline is not a vitamin or mineral in the traditional sense—it is an essential nutrient that the body produces in limited quantities and cannot synthesize in sufficient amounts for optimal function, making dietary and supplemental intake necessary for most people. Its role in fatty liver disease is mechanistically direct: The liver uses phosphatidylcholine—a choline-containing phospholipid—as the structural backbone of VLDL particles, the vehicles through which the liver exports accumulated fat into circulation. Without adequate choline, VLDL synthesis is impaired, fat export stalls, and triglycerides accumulate inside liver cells. Choline deficiency is a validated experimental model for inducing fatty liver, which makes it one of the most mechanistically foundational nutritional factors in MASLD.

The reason choline is so specifically important to the liver comes down to a single enzyme: PEMT (phosphatidylethanolamine N-methyltransferase). The liver has two ways to produce phosphatidylcholine—the phospholipid used to assemble VLDL particles. One uses dietary choline directly. The other, the PEMT pathway, synthesizes it internally using SAMe (S-adenosylmethionine) as a methyl donor. PEMT accounts for roughly 30 percent of the liver's phosphatidylcholine production—and critically, the phosphatidylcholine it produces is the preferred form for VLDL assembly. When PEMT activity is low, the liver cannot build enough VLDL export vehicles, triglycerides accumulate in hepatocytes, and steatosis follows regardless of how much fat the person is actually eating.[224]

PEMT activity is regulated in part by estrogen—which is why premenopausal women have a degree of natural protection against fatty liver that postmenopausal women lose. As estrogen declines after menopause, PEMT expression falls, the internal phosphatidylcholine synthesis pathway weakens, and dietary choline requirements rise precisely when many women are already consuming less. This is not a minor adjustment: Some research suggests postmenopausal women may need substantially more dietary choline than younger women to maintain the same degree of hepatic fat export.

A common genetic variant in the PEMT gene—present in a meaningful proportion of the general population—further reduces enzyme activity independent of estrogen or diet.[225] People carrying this variant are significantly more susceptible to fatty liver even on a diet that would be entirely adequate for someone without it. If you have lean MASLD, a family history of liver disease without obvious metabolic cause, or are postmenopausal with confirmed fatty liver, PEMT genetic testing through a direct-to-consumer service (23andMe or similar) or a functional medicine panel is worth discussing with your physician. The practical corrective is the same regardless of test result—prioritizing choline-rich foods and supplementing if intake is low—but knowing your genetic status sharpens the motivation considerably. PEMT also depends on SAMe as its methyl donor, which means adequate B12, folate, and B6 status are supporting conditions for the pathway to function well—providing one more reason why methylation-cycle nutrients appear repeatedly throughout the metabolic support framework in this book.

Some integrative practitioners also recommend prioritizing glutathione support—through NAC supplementation as discussed in this chapter; or direct S-acetyl glutathione supplementation—and antioxidant compounds that support superoxide dismutase (SOD) activity, such as zinc, copper, and manganese, for individuals with confirmed PEMT variants or postmenopausal women with MASLD. The reasoning is mechanistically sound: When liver fat export is impaired and triglycerides accumulate, the resulting oxidative stress depletes the liver's antioxidant defenses. Addressing the upstream cause through choline and methylation nutrients remains the primary strategy; antioxidant support is a reasonable secondary layer, particularly for those who have not yet normalized liver enzymes despite adequate choline intake. This specific application has not been studied in clinical trials targeting PEMT variants directly—it is an evidence-informed inference rather than a tested protocol, and worth discussing with a practitioner familiar with nutrigenomics.

Choline insufficiency is common in people with MASLD.[226] Dietary surveys consistently find that most adults consume well below the adequate intake of 425 mg (women) to 550 mg (men) per day. People eating low-egg, plant-forward diets are at particular risk. Postmenopausal women face amplified risk because estrogen normally upregulates the PEMT pathway—the body's internal choline synthesis route—and this pathway declines significantly after menopause, increasing dietary and supplemental requirements at precisely the age when MASLD risk is rising most steeply.

Epidemiological data shows consistent inverse associations between dietary choline intake and MASLD prevalence and severity. Dietary sources include egg yolks (the richest common source), liver, beef, shrimp, salmon, and legumes. For those with consistently low egg intake or documented insufficiency, supplemental choline bitartrate (250 to 500 mg/day) or the more bioavailable alpha-GPC form (300 to 600 mg/day) provides a practical corrective strategy. Choline is well-tolerated at these doses; very high doses—above 3,500 mg/day—can cause a fishy body odor, mild blood pressure reduction, and gastrointestinal symptoms, but these effects are well above standard supplemental ranges.

In light of research establishing choline insufficiency as a major driver of MASLD by impairing the liver's ability to export lipids,[227] recent epidemiological findings from the NHANES 2017-2020 dataset add a layer of complexity for those who already have the condition.[228]

The data indicates that while choline intake is not significantly associated with the initial prevalence of MASLD, higher intake among individuals with existing MASLD is linked to significantly higher odds of developing liver fibrosis. This association was particularly pronounced in men and individuals with metabolic risk factors like central obesity, suggesting that while the nutrient is essential to prevent fat accumulation, high levels may paradoxically contribute to disease progression in certain vulnerable subsets.

The form of choline is a significant factor in how the body processes it and how it might influence liver health. The NAHANES data primarily evaluated total choline intake rather than delineating choline intake by form. Different forms of choline are metabolized differently by gut bacteria. Forms like choline bitartrate or those found in certain foods can be converted by gut microbiota into trimethylamine (TMA), which the liver then converts to TMAO (trimethylamine N-oxide). High TMAO levels are associated with increased inflammation and cardiovascular risk. Alpha-GPC is a phospholipid-related form that can effectively deliver choline for the liver to produce phosphatidylcholine and the VLDL-exporting pathways, potentially bypassing some of the gut-mediated TMAO production compared to free choline salts. This suggests that alpha-GPC is lower risk, but total choline intake and the metabolic byproduct (TMAO) are critical factors to monitor when consuming supplemental choline.

Tier 2: Promising Natural Compounds with Meaningful Evidence

The following supplements have a growing body of evidence—plausible mechanisms, positive clinical signals, and reasonable safety—but require more large-scale, high-quality human trials before they can be positioned with the same confidence as Tier 1 supplements. They are worth considering as part of a comprehensive protocol, particularly for their additive and overlapping mechanisms.

Silymarin (Milk Thistle)

Milk thistle extract—standardized to its active flavonolignan complex, silymarin—is the oldest and most extensively studied natural compound for liver health. Its use in liver disease dates to ancient Greek and Roman medicine, and the modern research base, while heterogeneous in quality, is substantial.

Silymarin acts as an antioxidant, stabilizes liver cell membranes against oxidative damage and toxin penetration, inhibits the pro-inflammatory NF-kB signaling pathway, and has shown anti-fibrotic properties by suppressing hepatic stellate cell activation—the cell type responsible for generating scar tissue in the liver.[229] Multiple clinical trials have documented improvements in ALT, AST, and GGT liver enzymes with silymarin supplementation, and several have shown reductions in liver fat and improvements in insulin resistance markers in individuals with MASLD.[230]

Bioavailability is the primary challenge with standard silymarin preparations—the compound is poorly absorbed from the gastrointestinal tract in conventional form. Phospholipid complex forms of silymarin (such as Siliphos or Silymarin Phytosome), in which silymarin is bound to phosphatidylcholine, show dramatically improved absorption—up to four to ten times greater than standard extracts.[231] A newer silymarin amino acid cocrystal (bound to proline) formulation also demonstrates enhanced bioavailability.[232] When choosing a milk thistle supplement, the form matters as much as the dose.

Standard dosing for conventional silymarin is 420 to 600 mg per day of a standardized extract (70 to 80 percent silymarin content). For phospholipid complex forms, lower doses are effective due to enhanced absorption. Silymarin is generally well-tolerated, with a mild laxative effect at high doses as the most common adverse effect.

Curcumin

Curcumin is the primary bioactive polyphenol in turmeric, and it acts through a broad range of anti-inflammatory, antioxidant, and metabolic mechanisms directly relevant to fatty liver disease. It inhibits NF-kB and TNF-alpha—two central inflammatory mediators active in MASH.[233] It activates AMPK, improving insulin sensitivity and suppressing hepatic fat production.[234] It has antifibrotic properties and modulates the gut microbiome toward less pro-inflammatory compositions.[235]

Clinical trials in people with MASLD have shown reductions in liver fat, improvements in ALT and AST, reduced HOMA-IR, and lower inflammatory markers with curcumin supplementation over twelve to twenty-four weeks.[236] Meta-analyses consistently support these effects, with liver enzyme improvements being the most robust finding across trials.[237]

Like milk thistle, bioavailability is curcumin's central limitation—standard curcumin powder is poorly absorbed from the gut. Several enhanced-bioavailability forms have been developed and tested: A curcumin-essential oil complex, phospholipid-bound curcumin, nanoparticle form, and curcumin with fenugreek soluble fiber all show meaningfully improved absorption compared to unformulated curcumin.[238] When selecting a curcumin supplement, an enhanced-bioavailability form is not optional—it is the difference between a supplement that works and one that passes through largely unabsorbed. Effective doses depend on the formulation; always follow the manufacturer's guidance for the specific form being used.

Berberine and Curcumin Combined

It is worth noting that berberine and curcumin share and complement several mechanisms—both activate AMPK, both suppress NF-kB inflammation, and both improve gut microbiome composition. In some research settings, their combination produces additive effects greater than either alone.[239] For people building a supplement protocol around metabolic health and liver support, these two compounds work synergistically and are commonly used together by clinicians with expertise in integrative metabolic medicine.

Green Tea Extract (EGCG)

Epigallocatechin gallate (EGCG) is the primary bioactive catechin in green tea and one of the most studied polyphenols in liver research. It activates AMPK, inhibits *de novo* lipogenesis in the liver, reduces hepatic fat accumulation, and provides antioxidant protection specifically targeting the oxidative stress pathways active in MASH.[240] It also modulates the gut microbiome toward greater diversity and lower endotoxin-producing bacterial populations.[241]

Clinical trials have found improvements in liver enzymes, liver fat, and inflammatory markers with green tea extract supplementation in people with MASLD.[242] Two to three cups of brewed green tea daily delivers meaningful amounts of EGCG through a food source, which is the most elegant approach. Concentrated EGCG supplements provide higher doses—typically 400 to 800 mg per day—but come with a safety caveat: High-dose EGCG supplements have been associated with rare but documented cases of liver toxicity,[243] paradoxically making a supplement intended to support liver health potentially harmful at excessive doses. Doses above 800 mg EGCG per day are not recommended, and anyone with advanced liver disease should discuss green tea extract supplementation with their physician before use.

The practical guidance for most people: Drink green tea regularly as a food-based source of EGCG. Supplement cautiously and at moderate doses if higher intake is desired.

Resveratrol

Resveratrol is a polyphenol found in red grapes, red wine, blueberries, and mulberries that has attracted significant research interest for its SIRT1-activating and AMPK-modulating properties. In animal models, resveratrol consistently reduces liver fat, improves insulin sensitivity, and reduces hepatic inflammation.[244] Human trial results have been more variable, with some studies showing meaningful improvements in liver enzymes and metabolic markers and others showing modest effects.[245]

The most consistent human findings are in people with significant insulin resistance or metabolic syndrome, suggesting that resveratrol's benefits may be most pronounced in higher-risk populations. Bioavailability is variable and absorption is enhanced when resveratrol is taken with a fat-containing meal or in formulations paired with piperine (a black pepper extract). Standard doses studied in trials range from 150 to 1,000 mg per day. Resveratrol is well-tolerated at these doses, with mild gastrointestinal effects being the most common adverse response.

Artichoke Leaf Extract

Artichoke leaf extract, standardized for its cynarin and chlorogenic acid content, supports liver health primarily through its effects on bile flow and cholesterol metabolism. It stimulates bile production and secretion, improving the liver's ability to process and excrete fats and cholesterol.[246] It also has documented antioxidant and mild anti-inflammatory effects in hepatic tissue, and several clinical trials have found improvements in liver enzymes and lipid parameters with artichoke extract supplementation in people with mild to moderate liver dysfunction.[247]

Artichoke extract is most valuable for people whose fatty liver disease is accompanied by impaired bile flow or elevated total cholesterol and LDL—a common metabolic cluster in MASLD. It complements rather than overlaps with most of the other liver-supportive supplements and is well-tolerated at standard doses of 600 to 1,800 mg per day of standardized extract.

Cinnamon Bark Extract

Cinnamon supplementation has moderate evidence for improving insulin resistance and metabolic markers, particularly in people with type 2 diabetes, prediabetes, metabolic syndrome, or PMOS. Multiple meta-analyses of randomized controlled trials show that cinnamon can reduce HOMA-IR with pooled effect sizes that are modest but consistent—roughly 0.54 to 0.78 standard deviation improvement—and produce reductions in fasting blood glucose, fasting insulin, and HbA1c, typically most pronounced at doses of 1 to 3 grams per day over eight to twelve weeks or more.[248,249]

The active compounds in cinnamon—particularly cinnamaldehyde and proanthocyanidins—improve insulin receptor sensitivity and reduce post-meal glucose spikes through multiple pathways including slowing gastric emptying and improving GLUT4 transporter activity in muscle.[250] Cinnamon also shows modest lipid-improving effects and some evidence of anti-inflammatory activity.

Its effects are not as strong or as consistent as the top-tier options like berberine, myo-inositol, or omega-3s, but cinnamon ranks as a reasonable, low-cost adjunct with genuine supportive data. Ceylon cinnamon (*Cinnamomum verum*) is preferable to cassia cinnamon for supplemental use, as cassia contains higher levels of coumarin—a compound that can be toxic to the liver at high doses, which is a meaningful concern when the goal is liver health. Culinary use of cinnamon at normal cooking amounts is safe with either variety; the coumarin concern applies specifically to high-dose supplementation with cassia.

N-Acetyl Cysteine (NAC)

N-acetyl cysteine is the direct precursor to glutathione—the liver's primary endogenous antioxidant and the central molecule in its detoxification system. Oxidative stress is a well-established driver in the progression from simple steatosis to MASH and fibrosis: When the liver's antioxidant defenses are overwhelmed, reactive oxygen species damage cell membranes, mitochondria, and DNA, triggering the inflammatory cascade responsible for disease progression. NAC replenishes glutathione stores, directly restoring this antioxidant capacity.

Clinical trials in people with MASLD have shown only minor reductions in ALT and AST liver enzymes and improvements in liver histology with NAC supplementation; however, it improved oxidative, glycemic, and inflammatory markers.[251] Its hepatoprotective mechanism is well-established clinically—NAC is the standard medical treatment for acetaminophen-induced liver toxicity, one of the most common causes of acute liver failure, which confirms its direct liver-protective action. Standard supplemental doses of 600 to 1,800 mg per day are well within a long-established safety record.

NAC is particularly relevant for two groups: people with elevated liver enzymes in the context of ongoing oxidative stress (MASH specifically), and anyone who uses acetaminophen regularly for pain management—since acetaminophen depletes hepatic glutathione, and the MASLD liver has diminished antioxidant reserve to begin with. Divide daily doses across two to three administrations for best absorption. NAC should be used with caution by people with cystinuria (a rare kidney stone condition), and high doses may interfere with certain medications—discuss with your physician if you are taking nitrates or blood thinners.

Coenzyme Q10 (CoQ10)

Mitochondrial dysfunction is a central mechanism in MASLD—impaired mitochondrial fat oxidation is one of the primary reasons the liver accumulates fat rather than burning it. Coenzyme Q10 is an essential component of the mitochondrial electron transport chain, the machinery responsible for generating ATP from fatty acid oxidation, and a fat-soluble antioxidant specifically positioned in the mitochondrial membrane where oxidative damage from liver fat metabolism is most concentrated.

Clinical trials in people with MASLD and nonalcoholic steatohepatitis have shown reductions in ALT and AST and improvements in inflammatory markers with CoQ10 supplementation.[252,253] Its relevance extends beyond liver health to a specific large subgroup of people with MASLD: those taking statin medications for cardiovascular risk management. Statins—which block the same HMG-CoA reductase pathway used to synthesize both cholesterol and

CoQ10—deplete CoQ10 levels significantly. A significant proportion of people reading this book will be on statins. For them, CoQ10 supplementation addresses both a drug-induced deficiency and a mechanistically relevant mitochondrial support need simultaneously.

The ubiquinol form of CoQ10 (the reduced, active form) is considerably more bioavailable than the more common ubiquinone form—particularly in older adults whose conversion capacity declines with age. Effective doses in trials typically range from 100 to 300 mg per day of ubiquinol, taken with a fat-containing meal for absorption. CoQ10 is very well tolerated; mild gastrointestinal discomfort is the most common adverse effect at higher doses.

TUDCA (Tauroursodeoxycholic Acid)

TUDCA is a bile acid derivative that addresses a specific mechanism of liver cell injury not targeted by any other supplement in this chapter: endoplasmic reticulum (ER) stress.[254] The endoplasmic reticulum is the cellular organelle responsible for protein folding and lipid synthesis. In the MASLD liver, chronic fat overload and inflammatory signaling overwhelm the ER's capacity, triggering a cellular stress response that promotes hepatocyte (liver cell) death and fibrogenic signaling—directly driving progression from steatosis toward MASH and scarring.

TUDCA acts as a chemical chaperone that stabilizes protein folding in the ER and reduces this stress response. Human trials have shown improvements in liver enzyme levels, insulin sensitivity, and inflammatory markers with TUDCA supplementation.[255,256] It also supports bile flow and has emerging evidence for gut barrier integrity—making it relevant to the gut-liver axis discussed in Chapter 8.

TUDCA's mechanism is primarily additive to every other supplement in this chapter—it does not overlap with antioxidant pathways or AMPK activation, but augments insulin sensitization. It is most relevant for people with more advanced steatohepatitis, elevated liver enzymes despite other interventions, or those who have not responded fully to standard supplement protocols. Typical doses studied range from 500 to 1,750 mg per day in divided doses. TUDCA is generally well tolerated; consult your physician before use if you have advanced liver disease, gallstones, or are taking bile acid sequestrants.

Quercetin

Quercetin is a flavonoid found in onions, capers, apples, and berries that brings a mechanistically distinct contribution to a liver health supplement protocol: autophagy induction.[257,258] Autophagy—the cell's self-cleaning process by which damaged organelles and accumulated lipid droplets are broken down and recycled—is one of the liver's primary mechanisms for clearing excess fat. Impaired autophagy is an established feature of MASLD progression, and restoring it is an active target in pharmaceutical research. Quercetin activates autophagy pathways alongside its well-documented anti-inflammatory (NF-kB inhibition) and antioxidant effects, placing it in a mechanistically unique position among natural compounds.

Clinical trials specifically in people with MASLD have shown reductions in liver fat, ALT, AST, and inflammatory markers with quercetin supplementation over eight to twelve weeks.[259] Its evidence base is comparable to resveratrol—which is already in this chapter—and its autophagy-induction mechanism is more directly relevant to liver fat clearance than resveratrol's SIRT1 pathway.

Quercetin is found in meaningful amounts in a whole-food diet rich in onions, capers, apples, and dark berries—making food-based intake a reasonable first approach. For supplemental use, bioavailability is enhanced by pairing with vitamin C (which stabilizes quercetin in the gut) or using phytosome formulations. Typical supplemental doses studied in MASLD trials range from 500 to 1,000 mg per day. Quercetin is very well tolerated; it may mildly enhance the effects of blood thinners at high doses, which warrants monitoring if anticoagulants are being taken.

HORMONAL SUPPORT SUPPLEMENTS

As discussed in Chapter 7, hormonal imbalances—particularly declining sex hormones with age and thyroid dysfunction—are frequently underappreciated contributors to metabolic dysfunction in MASLD. Targeted supplementation can provide meaningful support alongside the lifestyle interventions that form the foundation of hormonal health.

For Men: Testosterone Support

Low testosterone is independently associated with higher visceral fat, worse insulin sensitivity, and elevated liver fat in men.[260] A meaningful proportion of men with MASLD have suboptimal testosterone levels—often undiagnosed—and addressing this is a legitimate part of a comprehensive metabolic strategy.

Several supplements have evidence-based support for naturally supporting testosterone levels and mitigating age-related hormonal decline in men:

- **Fenugreek (standardized to 50% saponins; branded forms include Fenutrax):** Fenugreek extract consistently shows modest improvements in free and total testosterone in clinical trials, likely through inhibition of aromatase (the enzyme that converts testosterone to estrogen) and 5-alpha reductase.[261] It also has direct metabolic benefits—improving insulin sensitivity and reducing fasting blood glucose—making it a particularly relevant supplement for men with MASLD and insulin resistance.[262] Take 500–600 mg in the morning before a meal, or 250–300 mg in the morning and before lunch. Allow 8 to 12 weeks before retesting testosterone levels.

- **Tongkat Ali (*Eurycoma longifolia*; LJ100 and Physta are clinically studied forms):** A Southeast Asian botanical with multiple clinical trials demonstrating improvements in free testosterone, reduced sex hormone-binding globulin (SHBG), improved body composition, and enhanced stress resilience.[263] Research suggests those with low testosterone who consume tongkat ali experienced a 37 percent increase in testosterone after 12 weeks. The LJ100 extract is the most rigorously studied standardized form. Take 200–400 mg in the morning or early day (may have mild stimulating effects; avoid late use to prevent sleep disturbance).
- **Ashwagandha (KSM-66 and Sensoril are the most clinically validated extracts):** An adaptogenic herb with strong evidence for lowering cortisol, improving body composition, and modestly improving testosterone levels in men under chronic stress—precisely the hormonal profile common in men with MASLD and metabolic syndrome.[264] Testosterone is increased on average 15 to 19 percent after

eight plus weeks of taking it.[265] Take 300–600 mg daily with food (to avoid stomach upset). It can be taken in the morning for energy and mood or in the evening for cortisol control and sleep support.

- **Shilajit (PrimaVie is a clinically studied purified form):** A purified mineral-rich resin compound from Himalayan rock formations with evidence for increasing free testosterone, improving mitochondrial function, and supporting energy metabolism. Ninety-day trials showed increases in total and free testosterone (20 percent and 19 percent respectively) and DHEA.[266] It is often combined with other male hormonal support supplements for additive effect. Take 500 mg daily in the morning on an empty stomach for better absorption.
- **Tesnor:** A plant-based food extract made from a proprietary blend of pomegranate peel (*Punica granatum*) and cocoa beans (*Theobroma cacao*); clinical research suggests that it works by stimulating the body's internal production of testosterone while simultaneously slowing down the process that converts testosterone into estrogen (aromatase inhibition). In studies involving both young and aging men, daily doses of 200 mg to 400 mg were found to significantly increase levels of free and total testosterone.[267] Beyond just the numbers on a blood test, men in these trials reported practical benefits such as improved muscle strength, increased libido, and a reduction in common "aging male symptoms" like fatigue and low mood. Take 200–400 mg in the morning after breakfast—400 mg produces faster and better results.

- **Diindolylmethane (DIM):** A compound derived from the breakdown of indole-3-carbinol in cruciferous vegetables. DIM acts as an aromatase inhibitor and shifts estrogen metabolism toward less potent estrogen metabolites—relevant for men with elevated estrogen from visceral fat-driven aromatization. Typical doses are 100–300 mg daily and should be taken in the morning to avoid sleep disturbance (possible stimulating effect).
- **Calcium D-glucarate (CDG):** Supports estrogen clearance through the glucuronidation pathway in the liver, helping to excrete excess estrogen that accumulates in men with high visceral fat. CDG also aids detoxification and is sometimes paired with DIM for additive effects. Take 500 mg up to three times daily with meals.
- **Supportive nutrients:** Zinc (15 to 50 mg elemental zinc), magnesium (400 mg; glycinate or malate forms for best absorption), vitamin B6 (10 mg), and vitamin D all serve as cofactors in testosterone synthesis and are commonly deficient in men with metabolic disease.

For Women: Hormonal Balance Support

Women experience a significant shift in fatty liver disease risk through the perimenopause and post-menopause transition, driven by declining estrogen and the accompanying shift in fat distribution toward visceral accumulation. Estrogen, progesterone, and testosterone don't just govern your menstrual cycle or manage menopause. They shape how your body handles insulin, where you store fat, and how readily your liver can clear metabolic waste. When these hormones fall out of balance—whether from perimenopause, PMOS, chronic stress, or simply the natural arc of aging—the liver often pays the price. Hormonal support for women with MASLD therefore centers on addressing estrogen imbalance—which, in most premenopausal and perimenopausal women, is a relative estrogen dominance pattern rather than estrogen deficiency—and supporting the transition through menopause with reduced metabolic disruption.

- **Diindolylmethane (DIM):** Supports healthy estrogen metabolism in women by promoting conversion of estrogens toward the 2-hydroxyestrone pathway—a less proliferative and more metabolically favorable estrogen metabolite—and away from the 16-hydroxyestrone pathway.[268] Particularly relevant for women with signs of estrogen dominance: heavy periods, premenstrual breast tenderness, weight gain in hips and thighs, or difficulty losing weight. Take 100–300 mg daily with food (better absorption) and in the morning to avoid interfering with sleep.
- **Calcium D-glucarate:** Works alongside DIM by inhibiting beta-glucuronidase, an enzyme produced by gut bacteria that can reactivate estrogens that the liver has already packaged for excretion—allowing them to be reabsorbed rather than cleared. Supporting estrogen clearance reduces the estrogen burden on the liver. Take 500 mg up to three times daily with meals.
- **Vitex (Chaste Tree Berry; Ze 440 and Agnucaston are clinically studied extracts):** Has the most evidence among botanicals for supporting progesterone relative to estrogen in the luteal phase, reducing PMS symptoms, and improving cycle regularity in premenopausal women with progesterone insufficiency—a common driver of estrogen dominance.[269] Vitex is a dopamine agonist that lowers

prolactin to reduce PMS, breast pain, irregular cycles, and some perimenopausal symptoms. Low doses of the standardized and clinically studied extracts can be taken (20–40 mg day in the morning during follicular phase or continuously), but higher doses of dried fruit extracts are necessary (100–200 mg) for effectiveness. It takes up to 12 weeks for full effects to be felt. Use cautiously in PMOS—may increase luteinizing hormone, which may be elevated in women with PMOS—or with dopamine-related meds.

- **Fenugreek (FenuSMART):** It might be surprising to find fenugreek on both the men's and women's hormone list, but here's what many people don't know: The standardization of a fenugreek extract determines what it actually does in your body. The same plant, processed differently, produces very different results for men versus women. FenuSMART is a clinically studied fenugreek extract standardized specifically for women's physiology. It contains a minimum of 10% protodioscin, at least 30% total saponins, and meaningful levels of trigonelline—a profile that directly targets female hormone pathways. Protodioscin is the key driver. It's a steroidal saponin that your body can convert into DHEA, a precursor hormone that supports both estrogen and testosterone production through normal metabolic pathways. Rather than introducing hormones from the outside, protodioscin essentially gives your hormone-producing glands better raw material to work with. Trigonelline adds another layer: It supports insulin sensitivity and helps modulate the androgen excess often seen in conditions like PMOS. It's also neuroprotective—say goodbye to brain fog—and mood-elevating. The research on FenuSMART is not based on folklore or tradition alone. Clinical trials have examined its effects on libido, hormonal markers, and sexual function in women—and the results are meaningful. In a double-blind, placebo-controlled trial published in Phytotherapy Research, women taking a standardized fenugreek extract showed significant improvements in sexual desire, arousal, and overall sexual function scores compared to placebo over 8 weeks.[270] Notably, these improvements correlated with measurable increases in free testosterone and estrogen levels, suggesting a genuine hormonal mechanism rather than a placebo response. Additional studies have found that this type of protodioscin-standardized extract supports menstrual regularity in women with irregular cycles and may reduce symptoms associated with hormonal imbalance, including fatigue, mood fluctuation, and low libido—all of which are more prevalent in women with underlying metabolic dysfunction.[271] For women in perimenopause or early menopause, the evidence suggests FenuSMART may help ease the transition by supporting the body's own hormone production during a period when that production becomes unpredictable. The clinically-effective dose is 500 to 600 mg daily, ideally with food, with most women experiencing noticeable changes within four to eight weeks.

- **Ashwagandha (KSM-66 and Sensoril):** Reduces cortisol, supports thyroid function, and modestly improves estrogen balance in perimenopausal women.[272] Particularly valuable for the stress-cortisol-metabolic dysfunction cycle that is common in middle-aged women managing MASLD. Ashwagandha helps stabilize the hypothalamic-pituitary-adrenal (HPA) axis to diminish the hormonal chaos that characterizes perimenopause. The common dosage is 300 to 600 mg per day, often in divided doses.

- **Rhaptontic rhubarb (Err 731):** Rhaptontic rhubarb (*Rheum rhaptontoicum*) shouldn't be confused with the culinary rhubarb from your grandmother's pie; it is a distinct species whose root contains powerful stilbene phytoestrogens—primarily rhaponticin and desoxyrhaponticin—that interact with estrogen receptors in a selective, tissue-specific way. Rhaponticin and desoxyrhaponticin are classified as selective estrogen receptor modulators (SERMs), naturally derived. They bind to estrogen receptors in specific tissues, providing estrogen-like signaling where it helps (the brain, bones, cardiovascular system) without stimulating breast or uterine tissue in the way that full estrogens do. In short, ERr 731 offers estrogen-like benefits in the tissues that need support—without the stimulatory effects that make women (and their doctors) cautious about phytoestrogens. This distinction matters enormously for safety, especially for women with a family history of hormone-sensitive cancers. ERr 731 is one of the most well-studied botanical extracts for menopausal symptoms, with multiple randomized, double-blind, placebo-controlled trials supporting its use. A landmark 12-week trial followed 109 perimenopausal women taking ERr 731 daily versus a placebo. The treatment group experienced a dramatic reduction in hot flash frequency and severity—

with some analyses showing a 70–73% reduction in symptom intensity—compared to modest changes in the placebo group.[273] The Menopause Rating Scale (MRS) and Kupperman Index both showed significant improvements across key menopausal domains: hot flashes, sleep disturbances, mood changes, and physical complaints. A 24-week extension study confirmed that these benefits persisted and continued to improve with longer use, without any adverse effects on breast tissue or endometrial thickness—findings that were confirmed by ultrasound.[274] Additional research has demonstrated that ERr 731 supports bone metabolism markers, suggesting a protective effect against the bone density loss that accelerates during menopause.[275] Cardiovascular markers, including LDL cholesterol and inflammatory cytokines, also trended favorably in some trials—a welcome connection for women managing both metabolic and menopausal health. This is different from soy isoflavones, which have weaker selectivity and a murkier safety record for women with breast cancer concerns.[276] Rhaptontic rhubarb has been studied specifically on breast cell lines and uterine tissue, and it has not shown stimulatory effects at clinical doses—a finding that has been independently replicated.[277]

- **Maca root (gelatinized):** Has evidence for improving hormonal symptoms in perimenopausal women—including mood, energy, libido, and hot flash frequency—through adaptogenic effects on the hypothalamic-pituitary axis rather than direct hormonal activity.[278] Red maca is often highlighted for female hormone balance, estrogen regulation, menopause support, and fertility. Yellow for general endocrine support; some blends (red-heavy) or specific phenotypes (e.g., Maca-GO) show stronger menopausal symptom relief. Black is used more for men and energy. Individual response varies. Take 1.5–3.5 grams daily in the morning or early afternoon (energizing for some; avoid late to prevent sleep issues) and allow 6 to 12 weeks of continuous use for full effects to be experienced. The typical dosage of Err 731 is only 4 mg daily with noticeable symptom improvements in four to eight weeks and full benefits seen at 12 weeks.

- **Black cohosh (Remifemin is the most studied standardized extract):** Specifically indicated for hot flashes, sleep disruption, and mood symptoms in menopausal women. Its mechanism remains debated but it is consistently effective for vasomotor symptoms (e.g., hot flashes and night sweats). Take 20–80 mg of standardized extract (most often 40 mg) daily in split doses with meals. Effects may start 2 to 4 weeks after use and peak at approximately 8 weeks.
- **Supportive nutrients:** Magnesium (400 mg; glycinate form is best tolerated), vitamin D, and omega-3 fatty acids (EPA and DHA) all support hormonal balance, sleep quality, and the metabolic parameters most relevant to MASLD in women.

A note on bioidentical hormones: For women with significant perimenopausal or postmenopausal symptoms that substantially impair quality of life or metabolic health, conversation with a physician about bioidentical hormone therapy—which can include topical progesterone cream (wild yam-derived) or prescription micronized progesterone—is appropriate. This is a clinical decision that extends beyond the scope of supplementation and requires individualized medical assessment. Hormonal decisions of this nature benefit enormously from working with a physician who has specific expertise in integrative or functional hormone medicine.

The connection between female hormonal status and liver health is more direct than many people realize. Estrogen, in healthy amounts, has a protective effect on the liver—it supports insulin sensitivity, reduces hepatic fat accumulation, and promotes anti-inflammatory signaling. As estrogen declines in perimenopause, the risk of MASLD rises sharply in women who were previously protected. Low testosterone in women is also associated with increased visceral fat and reduced lean muscle mass, both of which drive metabolic dysfunction.

Supporting the hormonal axis with a clinically standardized botanical (like FenuSMART or Vitex) isn't a cosmetic consideration—it's a metabolic one. Better hormonal balance means better insulin sensitivity, better body composition, and a more favorable environment for liver repair.

Here's where it gets especially relevant for this book. The metabolic changes of menopause—declining estrogen, rising visceral fat, worsening insulin resistance—are major drivers of MASLD progression in women over 45. It's no coincidence that MASLD rates in women jump significantly after menopause. Estrogen is a metabolic protector. When it declines, the liver loses some of its buffering capacity against fat accumulation and inflammation.

By supporting estrogen receptor signaling in a targeted way (like with ERr 731) it may help blunt some of the metabolic consequences of estrogen decline—not by replacing hormones, but by helping the body make better use of what it has. This makes it a genuinely relevant tool in a MASLD protocol for perimenopausal and postmenopausal women, not just a menopause-symptom management product.

THYROID SUPPORT

Thyroid dysfunction is significantly more common in people with fatty liver disease than in the general population, and its metabolic consequences—fatigue, impaired fat oxidation, weight gain, worsened insulin resistance—can undermine every other lifestyle intervention. When thyroid dysfunction is present and unaddressed, the ceiling on metabolic improvement is considerably lower than it should be.

For people with Hashimoto's thyroiditis (autoimmune hypothyroidism) or subclinical hypothyroidism, targeted nutritional support can meaningfully complement medical management:

- **Selenium (as selenomethionine, 200 mcg per day):** Selenium is essential for the conversion of the inactive thyroid hormone T4 to the active form T3, and for the antioxidant protection of thyroid tissue from the oxidative stress generated during hormone synthesis. Selenomethionine is the most bioavailable form. Multiple clinical trials have shown that selenium supplementation reduces thyroid antibody levels in individuals with Hashimoto's and modestly improves thyroid hormone conversion.[279] This is one of the most consistently evidence-supported nutritional interventions specifically for autoimmune thyroid disease.

- **Desiccated animal organ extracts (thyroid and liver):** Desiccated thyroid glandular supplements derived from bovine or porcine sources contain thyroid-specific peptides, cofactors, and trace nutrients that support thyroid cell function. While not equivalent to prescription thyroid hormone replacement, glandular thyroid supplements are commonly used in integrative medicine as supportive adjuncts. Commonly used supplements include: Allergy Research Group Thyroid Natural Glandular, Forefront Health Raw Desiccated Thyroid Glandular, and Ancestral Supplements Grass Fed Beef Thyroid. For people with mild subclinical hypothyroidism, they may provide meaningful support without the side effect profile of pharmaceutical thyroid medications.

For a more comprehensive discussion of natural approaches to thyroid health, including Hashimoto's thyroiditis and other autoimmune thyroid conditions, see the companion volume *Beating Autoimmune Thyroid Conditions Naturally* by this author.

How to Choose High-Quality Supplements

The supplement industry in most countries is not subject to the same pre-market regulatory scrutiny as pharmaceuticals. This means that the label on a supplement bottle does not guarantee that the product contains what it claims, at the dose it claims, without contaminants. Quality varies enormously between manufacturers, and this variability has real consequences for both efficacy and safety.

The following quality indicators narrow the field considerably:

- **Third-party testing and certification:** Look for products certified by NSF International, USP (United States Pharmacopeia), Informed Sport, or ConsumerLab. These organizations independently test supplements for label accuracy, potency, and the absence of heavy metals, pesticides, and undeclared adulterants. Certification is not mandatory, but its presence is a meaningful quality signal.

- **Clinically studied branded ingredients:** Many of the supplements discussed in this chapter have specific branded forms with their own clinical trial records—LJ100 for tongkat ali, KSM-66 for ashwagandha, BCM-95 for curcumin, PrimaVie for shilajit, Siliphos for silymarin. These are not merely marketing designations; they indicate that the specific form and concentration in the product is what was used in clinical research. Generic versions may or may not be equivalent.

- **Transparent labeling:** Reputable manufacturers list the full name of every ingredient, the dose of each active compound (not just the total blend weight), and the specific form of each ingredient. Proprietary blends that list combined ingredient weights without individual doses mean you cannot evaluate whether a dose is therapeutic or not.

- **Good Manufacturing Practice (GMP) certification:** GMP certification indicates that the manufacturing facility follows standardized quality control procedures. In the US, NSF GMP certification is the most rigorous; FDA-registered facilities meet a baseline but lower standard. EU-manufactured supplements are subject to stricter pre-market quality requirements than those manufactured in many other regions.

- **Avoid excessive proprietary "blends" with redundant ingredients:** Some products contain ten or more ingredients at sub-therapeutic doses—enough to list on the label but not enough to produce the documented benefits of any individual compound. A focused supplement with three to five high-quality ingredients at clinical doses is generally preferable to a sprawling formula with everything at trace amounts.

Interactions, Safety, and When to Ask Your Doctor

Most of the supplements in this chapter have favorable safety profiles when used at evidence-based doses in healthy adults. But certain combinations, health conditions, and medications warrant specific awareness.

- **Blood sugar-lowering medications:** Berberine, chromium, inositol, and cinnamon all have glucose-lowering effects. Combined with metformin, insulin, sulfonylureas, or GLP-1 agonists, they can produce additive effects that lower blood sugar further than intended. This is not a reason to avoid these supplements—it is a reason to monitor blood sugar more closely when adding them and to inform your prescribing physician.
- **Blood thinners (anticoagulants):** Omega-3 fatty acids, vitamin E, and some herbal supplements (including turmeric, ginger, and garlic in high doses) can have mild anticoagulant effects. People taking warfarin, clopidogrel, or newer anticoagulants should discuss supplement additions

with their physician and may require more frequent INR monitoring.

- **Cytochrome P450 interactions:** Berberine and some polyphenols interact with CYP3A4 and other liver enzymes that metabolize many common medications. If you are taking medications with narrow therapeutic windows—cyclosporine, certain statins, certain antiarrhythmics—discuss these interactions with your pharmacist or physician before adding berberine or high-dose polyphenol supplements.
- **Liver disease severity:** Some supplements that support healthy liver function can be harmful to a liver with severely compromised function. If you have advanced fibrosis, cirrhosis, or significantly elevated liver enzymes, supplement choices should be reviewed with the physician managing your liver care before use.
- **Pregnancy and breastfeeding:** Many supplements discussed in this chapter—including berberine, high-dose vitamin E, and several herbal adaptogens—are not established as safe in pregnancy or lactation. Pregnant or breastfeeding women should restrict supplementation to what is clearly established as safe in these contexts and should discuss any supplement use with their obstetric provider.

Start Here: Building Your Supplement Protocol

The following framework is designed to help you build a rational, evidence-based supplement protocol suited to your specific situation—rather than trying to take everything at once.

Step 1 – Address Deficiencies First

- Test your vitamin D level and supplement to bring it to 40 to 80 ng/mL if deficient
- Consider a high-quality omega-3 supplement (2 to 4 grams EPA/DHA daily) if fatty fish is not a regular part of your diet
- Assess magnesium status with an RBC magnesium test (not serum). If suboptimal—which is common in insulin-resistant individuals—supplement with 300 to 400 mg elemental magnesium as glycinate or malate daily. This is one of the lowest-risk, highest-yield additions available for people with insulin resistance.
- Evaluate your dietary fiber intake—if consistently below 20 grams per day, address this with food before adding supplements

Step 2 – Add Metabolic Support Based on Your Profile

- Significant insulin resistance, prediabetes, or MASLD with metabolic syndrome: Consider berberine (900 to 1,500 mg/day divided), inositol (2 to 4 g myo-inositol/day), or both
- Elevated liver enzymes with confirmed liver damage: Discuss vitamin E (800 IU/day) with your physician if you have biopsy-confirmed MASH and are nondiabetic; silymarin phospholipid complex is a reasonable adjunct with minimal risk
- Genetic pathway support: Niacinamide (250 to 500 mg/day) for the microRNA-93/SIRT1 pathway is a low-risk, low-cost addition

Step 3 – Layer in Liver-Supportive Compounds

- Silymarin (phospholipid complex or cocrystal form) for antioxidant liver cell membrane protection
- Curcumin (enhanced-bioavailability form) for anti-inflammatory and AMPK-activating effects
- Artichoke extract if bile flow and cholesterol are concerns

Step 4 – Address Hormonal Contributors If Relevant

- Men: Evaluate testosterone status; consider foundational supportive nutrients (zinc, magnesium, vitamin D) before botanical testosterone support
- Women: Evaluate estrogen dominance indicators; consider DIM and calcium D-glucarate if relevant; discuss perimenopausal hormonal support with a knowledgeable provider
- Everyone: Rule out thyroid dysfunction—particularly if fatigue and weight management resistance persist despite consistent lifestyle effort

> ***The Minimum Viable Supplement Protocol.*** *If you want to keep it simple, the combination with the strongest evidence-to-cost-to-risk ratio for most people with fatty liver disease is omega-3 fatty acids (2 to 4 g EPA/DHA daily), vitamin D (optimized to 40 to 60 ng/mL by testing), magnesium (300 to 400 mg glycinate or malate daily, particularly if RBC testing confirms suboptimal status), and berberine (900 to 1,500 mg/day with meals) or myo-inositol (2 to 4 g/day) if insulin resistance is a prominent feature. These three address the most central metabolic drivers*

> *of the disease through distinct, well-documented mechanisms. Everything else is additive.*

✦ ✦ ✦

Key Takeaways

- Supplements support lifestyle change—they do not replace it. Every supplement in this chapter works best when dietary, exercise, sleep, and gut health foundations are already in place.
- Tier 1 supplements with the strongest evidence for MASLD include omega-3 fatty acids (EPA/DHA), vitamin E (for nondiabetic MASH under medical guidance), vitamin B3 (niacinamide for the microRNA-93/SIRT1 pathway), berberine (AMPK activation, insulin sensitivity), vitamin D (optimize to 40 to 80 ng/mL), inositol (insulin signaling), chromium (insulin action support), and magnesium (insulin receptor function, sleep quality, inflammation—address deficiency with RBC testing rather than serum levels).
- Tier 2 compounds with meaningful but less definitive evidence include silymarin (liver cell membrane protection, anti-fibrotic), curcumin (anti-inflammatory, AMPK), green tea extract/EGCG (moderate doses only), resveratrol (SIRT1, AMPK), artichoke extract (bile flow, cholesterol), and cinnamon bark extract (modest insulin resistance benefit).
- Sex hormone support—testosterone-supporting compounds in men and estrogen-balancing compounds in women—addresses a frequently underdiagnosed contributor to metabolic dysfunction in MASLD, particularly in middle age and beyond.

- Thyroid support, particularly selenium as selenomethionine, is meaningful for people with Hashimoto's or subclinical hypothyroidism and should be addressed before concluding that lifestyle intervention has reached its ceiling.
- Quality matters enormously in supplement selection. Seek third-party tested products, clinically studied branded forms, and transparent labeling of individual ingredient doses.
- Build your protocol systematically: Address deficiencies first, add metabolic support based on your specific profile, layer in liver-supportive compounds, and address hormonal contributors if relevant. The minimum viable protocol—omega-3s, optimized vitamin D, magnesium, and berberine or inositol—covers the most central mechanisms for most people.

✦ ✦ ✦

With the evidence-based supplement landscape mapped, Chapter 10 turns to a complementary and often misunderstood category of natural support: essential oils. Positioned clearly as integrative tools rather than primary treatments, the chapter examines what the preclinical and early clinical evidence actually shows about their metabolic-supporting properties—and how they can be used practically and safely within a comprehensive liver health strategy.

CHAPTER 10

Essential Oils and Liver Health

Science, Skepticism, and Practical Integration

Essential oils occupy an unusual position in the health and wellness landscape. On one side, enthusiastic users attribute near-miraculous properties to them—cures, reversals, transformations. On the other side, skeptics dismiss them entirely as fragrant liquids with no meaningful biological effect. The truth, as it usually is, sits somewhere between these poles—and it is more interesting than either extreme suggests. As the most potent botanical extracts currently available, essential oils act as multitarget polypharmacological solutions that help the body perform its healing functions more effectively.

Plants have been producing bioactive chemical compounds for hundreds of millions of years. These compounds—the concentrated essence of which is what we call essential oils—evolved primarily as chemical defenses against bacteria, fungi, insects, and competing plant species. The same properties that make oregano oil an effective antimicrobial against gut pathogens and cinnamon bark oil a disruptor of fungal cell membranes developed for the plant's benefit primarily, and an argument could be made for humans secondarily.

They are real, they are documented, and they are increasingly the subject of serious scientific investigation.

This chapter approaches essential oils the way the rest of this book approaches every intervention: through the lens of what the evidence actually shows. Most of the research on essential oils and liver health is preclinical—conducted in cell cultures and animal models—and that limitation will be stated clearly wherever it applies. But preclinical evidence is not worthless. It identifies mechanisms, establishes plausibility, and provides the scientific rationale for human trials that are gradually accumulating. What is important is to not mistake "we have a plausible mechanism and promising early data" for "this is a proven treatment."

Used with appropriate expectations, essential oils offer genuine value as a complementary layer within a comprehensive liver health strategy. Not as the foundation—that remains diet, movement, sleep, stress management, and the gut-liver axis. But as a set of practical, accessible tools that can support stress reduction, digestive function, antimicrobial balance in the gut, and the anti-inflammatory environment that liver healing requires. That is a real and worthwhile role, honestly defined.

How Essential Oils Work: A Brief Mechanistic Overview

Essential oils are complex mixtures of volatile organic compounds—primarily terpenes, terpenoids, phenols, aldehydes, esters, and alcohols—extracted from plant material through steam distillation, hydrodistillation, or cold pressing. A single essential oil may contain dozens to hundreds of individual chemical constituents, each with its own biological activity, and the interactions between them often produce effects that no single compound produces alone.

Think of an essential oil as a chemical orchestra rather than a solo instrument. Cinnamon bark oil, for example, contains trans-cinnamaldehyde as its dominant active compound—but its full biological effect involves dozens of supporting constituents that modulate how cinnamaldehyde behaves in the body, improve its stability, and expand its range of activity. This complexity is both what makes essential oils scientifically interesting and what makes them difficult to study with the same precision as isolated pharmaceutical compounds.

At the cellular level, the bioactive compounds in essential oils interact with biological systems through several primary mechanisms, each relevant to fatty liver disease.

Anti-Inflammatory Mechanisms

Many essential oil constituents inhibit NF-kB—the master transcription factor that controls the expression of pro-inflammatory genes throughout the body and is one of the central drivers of the progression from simple fatty liver to MASH.[280] They also suppress the NLRP3 inflammasome, a protein complex that amplifies inflammatory signaling in response to cellular stress and metabolic damage. These are not minor or peripheral targets. NF-kB and the NLRP3 inflammasome are at the molecular heart of liver inflammation in MASLD, and their inhibition by plant-derived compounds is a biologically credible mechanism—not a vague claim about "reducing inflammation."

Terpenes—particularly monoterpenes like limonene (dominant in citrus oils) and sesquiterpenes like beta-caryophyllene (found in copaiba and black pepper essential oils)—have documented NF-kB inhibitory activity.[281] Beta-caryophyllene is particularly interesting because it is a selective agonist of the CB2 cannabinoid receptor,[282] which mediates anti-inflammatory effects in the liver and gut without the psychoactive effects of CB1 activation. This mechanism is supported by a growing body of pharmacological research.

Antioxidant Pathways

Oxidative stress—an excess of reactive oxygen species that damage liver cell membranes, mitochondria, and DNA—is a primary driver of MASH progression. Many essential oil constituents are potent antioxidants that neutralize these reactive species before they trigger inflammatory cascades.[283]

The antioxidant activity of essential oils operates through two main pathways: direct free radical scavenging (the compound directly neutralizes a reactive oxygen species) and indirect activation of the Nrf2 pathway—the cell's master antioxidant defense system. Nrf2 activation upregulates the production of the body's own antioxidant enzymes (superoxide dismutase, catalase, glutathione peroxidase), creating a more sustained and comprehensive protective effect than direct scavenging alone. Several essential oil constituents—including citral (geranial + neral) in lemongrass, linalool from lavender, and certain phenolic terpenes—have demonstrated Nrf2-activating activity in hepatic cell lines.[284]

Lipid Metabolism and Insulin Signaling

A smaller but meaningful body of preclinical research documents effects of specific essential oil constituents on hepatic lipid metabolism and insulin signaling pathways. These include suppression of the key enzymes driving *de novo* lipogenesis (SREBP-1c and fatty acid synthase), activation of PPAR-alpha (which promotes fat oxidation in the liver), and improvements in insulin receptor sensitivity in hepatic and adipose cell models.[285]

These findings are primarily from *in vitro* and animal studies and have not been replicated at scale in human clinical trials. They establish biological plausibility and provide a scientific rationale for the dietary use of the relevant plant foods—but they do not, at this stage, justify treating essential oil supplementation as equivalent to the dietary and metabolic interventions discussed in earlier chapters.

ESSENTIAL OILS WITH RELEVANCE TO FATTY LIVER: THE EVIDENCE

The following oils have the most directly relevant preclinical evidence for fatty liver disease and its metabolic drivers. Each entry is clear about the level of evidence available and what it does—and does not—tell us.

Ginger Essential Oil

Ginger (*Zingiber officinalis*) is among the most studied plant-derived compounds in MASLD research,[286] and its essential oil contains concentrated amounts of key bioactive constituents, like the sesquiterpenes alpha-zingiberene, beta-sesquiphellandrene, and *ar*–curcumene. Research found that ingestion of ginger essential oil prevented the progression of nonalcoholic steatohepatitis in a mouse model by blocking the NLRP3 inflammasome and remodeling the gut microbiota and the LPS-TLR4 inflammatory pathway—two of the most critical mechanisms in MASH progression discussed in Chapters 2 and 8.[287] The oil reduced liver damage, inflammation, and fat buildup primarily by improving gut health and reducing harmful substances (bacterial toxins) that reach the liver. Based on this, ginger shows promise as a natural supplement that could help prevent of slow down liver disease.

These are mouse model findings, not human clinical trials. But the mechanism—NLRP3 and TLR4 inhibition alongside gut microbiome modulation—is directly relevant to human fatty liver disease biology, and the culinary use of ginger (both fresh root and the essential oil used in cooking) is well-supported by this mechanistic evidence. Ginger essential oil can be used aromatically, topically over the abdomen when diluted appropriately, and in a capsule or softgel when a pure, high-quality oil is available.

Garlic Essential Oil

Garlic's (*Allium sativum*) therapeutic reputation is ancient, and modern science has given it a reasonable evidence base. It's essential oil is not common, but it does exist, and concentrates the bioactive sulfur compounds in the bulb. Research reported that garlic essential oil protected against obesity-triggered fatty liver disease through modulation of lipid metabolism and oxidative stress pathways in an animal model.[288] Allicin is a primary active compound in garlic that possess multiple medicinal properties, but lesser known is the medicinal value of its transformation products, including diallyl disulfide and diallyl trisulfide. They are released when garlic is crushed or processed, including when it is distilled to produce an essential oil. These compounds are well-researched and have demonstrated anticancer, cardioprotective, immunomodulatory (balancing or adjusting how your immune system responds), liver protective, kidney protective, neuroprotective, and anti-fatty liver properties.[289]

Of particular relevance to the gut-liver axis discussion in Chapter 8: Garlic-derived organosulfur compounds show selective antimicrobial activity against the gram-negative dysbiotic bacteria and *Candida* species that produce endogenous ethanol in the gut.[290,291] The garlic in a well-constructed Mediterranean-style diet is not merely flavoring—it is, among other things, a gentle and continuous modulator of the microbial environment in the gut.

The difficulty in using garlic essential oil is first its limited availability. Secondly, it is very irritating to the skin and a highly potent aroma, limiting its use topically and aromatically. It can be placed in an empty veggie capsule with lots of olive oil and consumed, but note that you are likely to smell of garlic after consuming it.

Sweet Orange Essential Oil

Sweet orange essential oil (*Citrus sinensis*) is composed predominantly of d-limonene—a monoterpene with documented anti-inflammatory, antioxidant, and lipid-modulating properties.[292,293] Research found that sweet orange essential oil protected against the formation of fatty liver in a high-fat diet animal model, with histological evidence of reduced hepatic steatosis and lower lipid peroxidation markers in treated animals.[294] The most remarkable finding of this animal model was that simply inhaling the essential oil reduced fat accumulation in liver cells.

Sweet orange activates PPAR-alpha—the nuclear receptor that promotes hepatic fat oxidation and is one of the targets of omega-3 fatty acids described in Chapter 9—and has demonstrated cholesterol-lowering effects through upregulation of hepatic LDL receptor expression. Citrus essential oils are also among the most extensively studied for their anxiolytic (anxiety-reducing) effects in human trials, making sweet orange a particularly practical choice for aromatic use targeting the stress-cortisol-liver pathway discussed in Chapter 7.

Sweet orange essential oil is one of the gentlest and most accessible oils for aromatic and topical use. It is well-tolerated, widely available, and inexpensive. The primary safety consideration is photosensitivity: Cold-pressed citrus oils (as opposed to steam-distilled) contain furanocoumarins that can cause skin sensitization when applied topically before sun exposure. Steam-distilled sweet orange oil avoids this concern. It can also be ingested in a capsule or softgel.

Anise Essential Oil

Anise essential oil (*Pimpinella anisum*), dominated by trans-anethole, has a smaller but targeted evidence base. Research examined its effects in a rat model of nonalcoholic fatty liver disease and documented reductions in liver fat accumulation and improvements in hepatic biochemical markers.[295] Ingestion of the oil reversed increased total cholesterol, LDL, and triglycerides and a decrease in HDL, showing it restores healthy lipid profiles. The oil also reduced liver enzymes and oxidative stress. Trans-anethole has demonstrated anti-inflammatory and antioxidant properties in multiple research settings, and its estrogenic-like activity may be relevant to the hormonal contributors to MASLD discussed in Chapter 7.

Anise essential oil is most practically used in a capsule and as a flavoring component. It pairs well with other digestive-supportive oils and has a long traditional use history for upper digestive complaints—bloating, gas, and sluggish digestion—that are common in people with dysbiosis and impaired gut motility.

ESSENTIAL OILS WITH RELEVANCE TO INSULIN SENSITIVITY

Insulin resistance is the central metabolic driver of fatty liver disease, and several essential oils have preclinical and limited clinical evidence for supporting insulin signaling pathways.

Cinnamon Bark Essential Oil

The essential oil of cinnamon bark (*Cinnamomum zeylanicum*) is one of the most studied for metabolic effects and connects directly to the supplement discussion of cinnamon extract in Chapter 9. Cinnamon bark oil is dominated by trans-cinnamaldehyde—the same compound responsible for cinnamon's characteristic aroma—which has demonstrated the ability to help the body respond better to insulin by increasing the activity of a protein called GLUT4, which helps move sugar into cells, and by improving how insulin signals in the body, based on studies in cells and animals.[296] Research has documented antidiabetic effects of cinnamon oil in both *in vitro* and diabetic animal models, with improvements in fasting blood glucose and insulin sensitivity markers.[297] Additionally, there was a noticeable drop in important health markers like blood sugar-related C-peptide, triglycerides, total cholesterol, and waste products in the blood. At the same time, HDL increased significantly, indicating better overall metabolic health.

Cinnamon bark essential oil also has potent antimicrobial activity—particularly against *Candida* species and gram-negative dysbiotic bacteria—making it one of the most mechanistically versatile oils in the context of MASLD.[298] The same properties that make it relevant to insulin signaling make it relevant to the endogenous ethanol-producing microbes discussed in Chapter 8. It is, in this sense, addressing two root causes through a single intervention.

An important safety distinction: Cinnamon bark oil is a potent skin sensitizer and mucous membrane irritant, particularly cinnamaldehyde. It must never be applied undiluted to the skin and requires a low dilution ratio (often 0.5 to 1 percent in a carrier oil) even for diluted topical application. It is suitable for direct oral ingestion only when encapsulated and properly mixed with an edible carrier oil.

Cumin Essential Oil

Cumin (*Cuminum cyminum*) essential oil has a specific and underappreciated evidence base for insulin resistance. A double-blind randomized placebo-controlled clinical trial evaluated ingestion of cumin essential oil in people with type 2 diabetes and found significant reductions in fasting blood glucose, insulin resistance markers, and serum inflammatory factors compared to placebo over twelve weeks.[299] The oil also reduced inflammatory markers (TNF-alpha and high-sensitivity C-reactive protein), which are increased in people with diabetes.

Another randomized, triple-blind human clinical trial evaluated ingestion of 75 mg of cumin essential oil three times daily in people with metabolic syndrome. The oil improved markers of metabolic syndrome and antioxidant activity and simultaneously decreased free radicals; therefore reducing oxidative stress.[300] This is human clinical trial data—a meaningfully higher level of evidence than the preclinical data available for most essential oils discussed in this chapter.

The primary active compounds in cumin oil—cuminaldehyde, gamma-terpinene, and beta-pinene—have antioxidant, anti-inflammatory, and glucose-modulating properties in cell and animal research settings.[301] Cumin is also among the most commonly used culinary spices in Mediterranean, Middle Eastern, and South Asian cuisines, meaning that its metabolic benefits are most naturally delivered through regular culinary use rather than supplemental application.

Based on the study doses, one to two drops are taken up to three times daily in a capsule for benefits.

Oregano Essential Oil

Oregano (*Origanum vulgare*) essential oil warrants discussion in two distinct contexts in this chapter: its anti-inflammatory and metabolic effects, and—connecting to the gut-liver axis discussion of Chapter 8—its antimicrobial activity against the specific dysbiotic organisms most implicated in fatty liver disease.

The primary bioactive constituent of oregano oil—carvacrol—has potent and well-documented antimicrobial activity against gram-negative bacteria, including several ethanol-producing species associated with MASLD, as well as against *Candida* and other dysbiotic yeasts.[302] This selectivity, combined with evidence of relative sparing of beneficial *Lactobacillus* and *Bifidobacterium* species at moderate doses, makes oregano oil one of the most mechanistically rational antimicrobial tools for gut dysbiosis in the context of fatty liver disease. Think of it as a scalpel rather than a sledgehammer—targeting the harmful fermenters while leaving the beneficial microbiome relatively intact, in a way that broad-spectrum antibiotics do not.

Carvacrol also demonstrates PPAR-alpha activating effects in cell models—the same fat-oxidation-promoting mechanism shared by omega-3 fatty acids—and anti-inflammatory activity through NF-kB inhibition.[303] The overlap between its antimicrobial and metabolic mechanisms makes oregano oil one of the most functionally relevant oils in a MASLD-specific protocol.

Safety considerations are important with oregano oil. It is among the most potent essential oils available and should never be used undiluted topically. For oral use, it must be a specifically labeled food-grade or therapeutic-grade product at a very low dilution—one to three drops in a capsule with diluted in a carrier oil. Oregano oil is not appropriate during pregnancy.

ESSENTIAL OILS FOR STRESS REDUCTION AND METABOLIC SUPPORT

Chapter 7 established that chronic stress and cortisol elevation are direct biological contributors to fatty liver disease—not merely behavioral influences on lifestyle choices, but hormonal forces that independently worsen insulin resistance, visceral fat accumulation, and liver inflammation. This is where aromatherapy has its most clinically credible human evidence base, and where the practical case for essential oils in a MASLD management strategy is strongest.

Lavender

Lavender essential oil (*Lavandula angustifolia*) has the most extensive human clinical evidence of any essential oil in the context of stress reduction and anxiety. Multiple randomized controlled trials have documented reductions in salivary cortisol, improvements in subjective stress and anxiety scores, reduced heart rate variability measures of sympathetic activation, and improved sleep quality with lavender aromatherapy.[304] It also has extensive evidence for anxiety and mood improvement when ingested.[305] The primary active compound, linalool, interacts with GABA-A receptors—the same receptor system targeted by benzodiazepine medications—to produce a calming, anxiolytic effect through inhalation.[306]

For someone managing fatty liver disease, lavender aromatherapy is one of the most accessible and lowest-risk tools for activating the parasympathetic nervous system during stressful periods. Diffusing lavender in the hour before sleep, applying a diluted blend to the wrists or back of the neck during high-stress periods, or using a lavender-infused sleep pillow spray are all practical delivery methods with documented cortisol-reducing effects. Ingesting it in a capsule—two drops, twice daily—sustains this benefit.

Bergamot

Bergamot (*Citrus bergamia*) essential oil, pressed from the rind, combines the anxiolytic properties of its linalool content with the mood-elevating and cortisol-modulating effects of its limonene and linalyl acetate constituents. Human trials have found meaningful reductions in anxiety and stress measures with bergamot aromatherapy in clinical settings.[307] It is one of the most commonly used essential oils in evidence-based aromatherapy practice precisely because of this combination of calming and uplifting effects.

The same photosensitivity caution that applies to sweet orange applies to bergamot: Bergapten-free (FCF—furanocoumarin-free) bergamot oil is the appropriate choice for topical use and should still be used cautiously, because, ironically, bergapten-free doesn't really mean free of bergapten, but reduced levels. Aromatic use carries no photosensitivity risk.

Frankincense

Frankincense (*Boswellia* spp.) contains terpenoids and incensole acetate that activates a specific protein called TRPV3.[308] When activated in the brain, TRPV3 plays a role in mood regulation. Incensole acetate reduced anxiety and depression-like behaviors in mice, suggesting it may help regulate emotions and elucidate the biological basis of the calming effects of incense.

Frankincense is most practically used aromatically for its grounding, calming, and meditative-enhancing effects—making it a valuable support for the mindfulness and breathing practices described in Chapter 7. It also has a long traditional use history for digestive complaints.

Peppermint

Peppermint (*Mentha × piperita*) essential oil's primary active compound, menthol, has well-documented effects on gastrointestinal function—reducing smooth muscle spasm, improving gallbladder contraction and bile flow, and alleviating bloating, gas, and nausea.[309] Enteric-coated peppermint oil capsules are actually recommended by some gastroenterological guidelines for irritable bowel syndrome, representing one of the clearest crossover points between traditional essential oil use and mainstream clinical practice.[310]

For people with fatty liver disease, particularly those experiencing the bloating, sluggish digestion, and upper right abdominal discomfort that can accompany impaired bile flow and gut dysbiosis, peppermint has practical and evidence-supported digestive utility. Aromatic or internal use also has documented effects on alertness, cognitive function, and exercise performance—making it a useful accompaniment to the morning exercise habit recommended throughout this book.

Lemon

Lemon (*Citrus limon*) essential oil, like other citrus oils, is dominated by d-limonene. Its relevance in a liver health context includes the PPAR-alpha activating and antioxidant effects described under sweet orange, along with documented mood-elevating and stress-reducing properties in human trials.[311,312] Lemon aromatherapy has been shown to reduce cortisol and improve mood in clinical studies,[313] and is one of the most practically accessible and broadly applicable oils for daily aromatic use.

Lemon oil is also one of the oils most commonly added to water in wellness contexts. A clarification worth making: Adding lemon essential oil to water is not the same as adding fresh lemon juice. Essential oil is hydrophobic and does not disperse in water—it floats on the surface and is consumed in concentrated form with each sip rather than evenly distributed. If using essential oil in water, it must be a therapeutic product specifically intended for internal use, and a drop in a full glass of water is the appropriate starting point.

Rosemary

Rosemary (*Salvia rosmarinus*) essential oil contains 1,8-cineole (eucalyptol), camphor, and alpha-pinene—compounds with documented anti-inflammatory and antioxidant properties in preclinical settings.[314] It has been studied for cognitive enhancement and cortisol modulation through inhalation, and animal research has documented hepatoprotective effects from rosemary extract in models of chemical liver stress. The essential oil's stimulating, circulation-enhancing character also makes it a useful complement to morning physical activity, applied topically (diluted) to the limbs or diffused during exercise.

DELIVERY METHODS: HOW TO USE ESSENTIAL OILS EFFECTIVELY

The way an essential oil is delivered determines what it can and cannot do. Each route of administration has different pharmacokinetic properties—how the active compounds enter the body, how quickly they reach their targets, and what concentrations are achievable. Understanding this makes the difference between using essential oils intelligently and using them randomly.

Aromatic Use

Inhalation is the fastest route of administration and the one with the most human clinical evidence, particularly for stress reduction and mood effects. When essential oil molecules are inhaled, they travel through the olfactory nerve—the only sensory nerve with direct access to the limbic system, the brain's emotional and hormonal regulation center—producing immediate effects on cortisol, heart rate, and autonomic nervous system tone.

Aromatic use includes diffusion (using an ultrasonic or nebulizing diffuser in a room), direct inhalation from a personal inhaler stick or by cupping hands around a drop on the palms and breathing deeply, and passive exposure through a personal diffuser pendant or bedside application. For stress reduction, sleep support, and mood enhancement, aromatic use is the most practical and most evidence-supported delivery method.

Ultrasonic diffusers—which use water and vibration to create a fine mist—are the most practical for room diffusion. Nebulizing diffusers deliver a higher concentration of oil molecules without water dilution and are more appropriate targeted therapeutic aromatic sessions or larger rooms. Diffuse for thirty to sixty minutes at a time rather than continuously, particularly in smaller spaces, to avoid olfactory fatigue.

Topical Use

Applying essential oils to the skin, properly diluted in a carrier oil, allows the active compounds to absorb transdermally and enter local circulation. Topical application over the abdomen (for digestive and liver-area applications), the back of the neck and temples (for stress and cortisol support), and the soles of the feet (a relatively nonsensitive surface appropriate for many oils) are the most common practical approaches.

Dilution is non-negotiable for safe and effective topical use. Essential oils are highly concentrated—it takes a large quantity of plant material to produce even a small volume of oil—and direct skin contact without dilution can cause sensitization and irritation, especially in people with a dysregulated immune system (autoimmune disease, eczema, allergies, etc.). The appropriate dilution for most adults is 4 to 10 percent essential oil in a carrier oil: roughly 24 to 60 drops of essential oil per 30 mL (one ounce) of carrier. Common carrier oils include fractionated coconut oil (odorless, light, and long shelf life), jojoba oil (technically a liquid wax, very skin-compatible), sweet almond oil, and castor oil. For potentially sensitizing oils—cinnamon bark, oregano, thyme, clove—a 0.5 to 3 percent dilution is more appropriate.

> ***Dilution Quick Reference.*** *1% dilution = 6 drops essential oil per 30 mL carrier oil | 2% dilution = 12 drops per 30 mL | 3% dilution = 18 drops per 30 mL | For potentially irritating oils (cinnamon bark, oregano, clove, thyme): 0.5% = 3 drops per 30 mL. Always perform a patch test on a small area of skin and wait 24 hours before broader application of any new oil.*

Oral Use

Oral use of essential oils is the most contested and most frequently misunderstood delivery method. Some essential oils, at appropriate dilutions and from pure, high-quality sources, have genuine utility for a variety of health concerns. Others (e.g., pennyroyal, sage CT thujone) are potentially harmful when ingested, making unsupervised oral use inappropriate.

The key principle is that not all essential oils are safe for oral use, and food-grade or therapeutic-grade labeling does not automatically make any dose or application safe. Essential oils that are generally recognized as safe (GRAS) for flavoring use by the FDA—including peppermint, ginger, lemon, orange, and cinnamon bark in flavoring quantities—have a different safety profile than the same oils taken in larger amounts as supplements. Fortunately, we have multiple clinical trials and decades of clinical experience that can help guide this use.

For the specific application of gut antimicrobial support relevant to fatty liver disease, enteric-coated peppermint oil capsules (for IBS and digestive symptoms) and oregano oil capsules (for targeted microbial rebalancing) are the most clinically supported oral approaches. Both should be used at labeled doses, for defined periods, and with awareness that even these well-studied applications warrant caution in people with significant liver disease, where the liver's metabolic processing of concentrated essential oil constituents may be impaired.

When in doubt about oral use of any specific essential oil, consult with a qualified aromatherapist, naturopathic doctor, or integrative medicine physician. The potential benefits of oral essential oil use for fatty liver disease do not, at this stage of the evidence base, justify taking significant risks with an already stressed liver.

Safety Considerations: What the Enthusiasm Sometimes Omits

Essential oils are powerful concentrated plant compounds, and power in biology is never one-directional. The same properties that make a compound bioactive make it capable of causing harm at inappropriate doses or in vulnerable populations. The following considerations apply to anyone using essential oils in the context of liver disease.

- **Liver disease severity and essential oil metabolism:** The liver is the primary site of essential oil constituent metabolism. In people with significantly compromised liver function—advanced fibrosis, cirrhosis, or severely elevated liver enzymes—the capacity to process and clear essential oil compounds is reduced. What is well-tolerated by a healthy liver may accumulate to problematic levels in a compromised one. People with advanced liver disease should discuss any essential oil supplementation or extended oral use with their hepatologist before proceeding.

- **Drug interactions:** Several essential oil constituents inhibit CYP450 liver enzymes—the same enzyme family responsible for metabolizing many common medications. Bergamottin from bergamot, furanocoumarins from other citrus oils, and certain phenolic compounds can slow the metabolism of drugs including statins, certain blood pressure medications, immunosuppressants, and anticoagulants. This is the same interaction pathway as grapefruit juice, which is better known as a drug interaction concern. If you are taking medications metabolized by CYP3A4 or CYP1A2, discuss essential oil use with your pharmacist or an informed practitioner. For discussion points review Appendix G in this author's book *Medicinal Essential Oils: The Science and Practice of Evidence-based Essential Oil Therapy.*

- **Pregnancy and breastfeeding:** Many essential oils are contraindicated during pregnancy due to their effects on uterine tone, hormone activity, or potential fetal toxicity. Oregano, cinnamon bark, thyme, and several others are generally considered inappropriate for use during pregnancy. Gentle oils like lavender, frankincense, and lemon are more widely considered safe in normal aromatic use during pregnancy, but erring toward conservatism and seeking guidance from a qualified practitioner is appropriate.

- **Children and infants:** Children metabolize essential oil compounds differently from adults and are significantly more sensitive to concentrated compounds. Several oils considered safe for adults—including eucalyptus, peppermint, and rosemary—warrant caution around or on infants and young children due to their menthol and 1,8-cineole content, which can cause respiratory distress. Always research pediatric safety guidelines specifically when using essential oils around children.

- **Quality and adulteration:** The essential oil market, like the supplement market, is rife with poor-quality and adulterated products. Adulterated, diluted, or synthetic essential oils are common in low-price products. For therapeutic use, look for oils from companies that provide GC/MS (gas chromatography/mass spectrometry) testing reports—documents that confirm the chemical constituents and their proportions, which establish both identity and purity. Third-party testing is the essential oil equivalent of supplement certification. Avoid oils that are implausibly inexpensive for the plant material required to produce them.

Putting It Together: A Practical Integration Framework

The most useful way to think about essential oils in a MASLD management strategy is through the lens of where they add practical value with low risk—and to be honest about where the evidence does not yet support more ambitious claims.

Highest-Value Applications (Best Evidence, Lowest Risk)

- **Stress and cortisol reduction (aromatic):** Lavender, bergamot, sweet orange, and frankincense through inhalation or diffusion. This is the application with the most human clinical evidence and directly addresses one of the root causes of fatty liver disease. Two to three aromatic sessions per day—morning, afternoon, and before sleep—is a practical starting point.

- **Sleep support (aromatic):** Lavender diffused in the bedroom or applied diluted to a sleep pillow. Supports the circadian alignment and sleep quality optimization discussed in Chapter 7.
- **Digestive support (aromatic and diluted topical):** Peppermint, ginger, and anise for bloating, gas, and post-meal digestive discomfort. Diluted topical application over the abdomen in a clockwise direction (following the direction of intestinal transit) is a traditional and practically reasonable application. Or, add a few drops total to a capsule with an edible carrier oil.
- **Culinary use of relevant oils and their source plants:** Garlic, ginger, cinnamon, cumin, and oregano deliver the bioactive compounds of their essential oils in a safe, food-integrated, and genuinely therapeutic form. Using these herbs and spices abundantly in cooking is not merely flavoring—it is a meaningful contribution to the antimicrobial, anti-inflammatory, and insulin-sensitizing interventions the research supports. If you need greater support add up to three drops total of these oils to a size 0 capsule and fill the rest of the capsule with an edible carrier oil.

Moderate-Value Applications (Promising Preclinical Evidence, Limited Human Data)

- **Gut antimicrobial support (diluted oral, with caution):** Oregano oil in enteric-coated capsules for targeted support against dysbiotic gut bacteria and yeasts. Use under the guidance of a knowledgeable practitioner, for defined periods, and not as a substitute for the dietary changes that address dysbiosis at its source.

- **Topical liver area application:** Diluted blends containing ginger, sweet orange, or frankincense applied over the right upper abdomen. The evidence for transdermal delivery of these compounds to hepatic tissue is limited, but the application is low-risk and the aromatic benefit of the practice itself (via inhalation during application) is real.
- **Exercise and morning energy support (aromatic):** Peppermint and rosemary diffused or inhaled before or during exercise have documented effects on alertness, perceived effort, and physical performance—supporting the consistent exercise habit that is foundational to liver health.

> ***The Right Frame for Essential Oils in This Protocol.*** *Essential oils work best when they are reinforcing and supporting what the rest of your lifestyle program is already doing—not when they are asked to do the heavy lifting alone. Lavender that helps you sleep better amplifies the metabolic benefits of good sleep. Peppermint that eases digestive discomfort makes dietary changes more tolerable and sustainable. Oregano that modestly shifts the gut microbial environment adds a layer of support to the dietary changes already reducing the fermentation substrate. That compounding, supporting role is genuinely valuable. It is also distinct from treatment—and keeping that distinction clear is what allows you to benefit from these tools without being misled by them.*

Key Takeaways

- Essential oils are concentrated bioactive plant compounds with real, documented mechanisms—including NF-kB inhibition, NLRP3 inflammasome suppression, Nrf2-mediated antioxidant activation, and selective antimicrobial activity. Most of the evidence is preclinical, and their role in a MASLD strategy is complementary support, not primary treatment.
- For fatty liver disease specifically, the oils with the most directly relevant preclinical evidence are ginger (NLRP3 inhibition, gut microbiome remodeling), garlic (lipid metabolism, antimicrobial against ethanol-producing gut bacteria), sweet orange (PPAR-alpha activation, antioxidant), and anise (hepatoprotective in animal models).
- For insulin sensitivity, cinnamon bark oil (GLUT4 activation, Candida and dysbiotic bacteria inhibition), cumin oil (human clinical trial evidence for glucose and insulin improvement), and oregano oil (carvacrol's PPAR-alpha and NF-kB activity plus targeted antimicrobial action) have the most relevant evidence.
- Aromatic use has the strongest human clinical evidence—particularly lavender, bergamot, and citrus oils for cortisol reduction, anxiety, and sleep support—and directly addresses the stress-cortisol-liver inflammation pathway established in Chapter 7.
- Culinary use of garlic, ginger, cinnamon, cumin, and oregano delivers their bioactive compounds in the safest and most integrated form, but more concentrated therapeutic support can be achieved via capsules. Abundant use of these foods in

everyday cooking is a genuinely therapeutic and low-risk application of essential oil science.

- Safety requires consistent attention: proper dilution for topical use (4 to 10 percent for most oils, 0.5 percent for potent sensitizers), caution with oral use, awareness of CYP450 drug interactions, consideration of liver disease severity, and third-party tested quality products.
- The practical integration hierarchy—aromatic stress and sleep support first, culinary use of relevant plants second, diluted topical application third, cautious targeted oral use under appropriate guidance fourth—positions essential oils as they deserve to be: a genuine complementary layer, intelligently used.

With the integrative and supplemental layers of the strategy now complete, Chapter 11 turns to the pharmaceutical landscape—the medications currently available for fatty liver disease, what they actually do, and how to think about them as part of a comprehensive approach that keeps lifestyle firmly in the primary role.

CHAPTER 11

Medications

What Works, What Doesn't, and Why the Conversation Matters

Here is a scenario that plays out in clinics regularly. A person is diagnosed with fatty liver disease and leaves with a referral and a recommendation to lose weight. They return six months later having made genuine lifestyle changes. The doctor notes the improvement and says: "Keep doing what you're doing." That is often the right advice.

But sometimes the picture is more complicated. The liver enzymes are not normalizing. The fibrosis markers are not moving in the right direction. The disease has progressed despite sincere effort. Or the person has diabetes, cardiovascular disease, or another metabolic condition that requires pharmaceutical or nutraceutical management alongside the liver disease. Or they want to understand the full landscape of options before deciding what role, if any, medication should play in their strategy.

Those are the people this chapter is written for. Not to promote medications, and not to discourage them—but to provide an honest, complete, and accessible account of what is currently available, what the evidence shows, and how to think about these tools in relation to the lifestyle foundation that this book has built.

The central message of this chapter is the same as it has been throughout: Medications support lifestyle, they do not replace it. No drug currently approved or in development addresses all the root causes of fatty liver disease simultaneously; and drugs should primarily be used when the benefit clearly outweighs the risks. The most effective outcomes consistently come from a combination approach in which lifestyle change is the primary intervention and medication, where appropriate, provides additional support. But "additional support" from the right medication, in the right person, at the right stage of disease, can be genuinely meaningful—and understanding the options is part of making informed decisions with your care team.

If your goal is to manage MASLD completely naturally, you can skip this chapter and move directly to Chapter 12. However, if you want to be prepared to have informed discussions with your healthcare provider, including why medication may not be appropriate in your case, this chapter is important to read.

It is worth stating plainly at the outset: The strategies in the preceding chapters—dietary change, regular movement, weight normalization, sleep, stress management, gut health, and targeted supplementation—are sufficient for the majority of people with early-stage fatty liver disease. Research consistently shows that meaningful lifestyle change produces measurable improvement in liver fat, insulin resistance, and metabolic markers in most people who implement it consistently. If you are reading this early in your MASLD journey, the most important thing you can do is not to find the right medication—it is to commit fully to the lifestyle and nutritional foundation this book has been building. Most people who do that will never need this chapter's content. For those who do reach this chapter's territory, it is here.

When Medications Enter the Picture

For most people with simple steatosis—early-stage fatty liver without significant inflammation or fibrosis—lifestyle intervention alone is appropriate first-line management, and medications are not routinely recommended by current guidelines. The liver at this stage is highly responsive to dietary change, exercise, weight loss, and the other interventions discussed in this book, and the risk-benefit calculation for adding pharmaceutical agents to an already-improving situation does not favor it.

The calculus begins to shift as the disease advances. Current guidelines from major hepatology societies consider medication more strongly in the following contexts:

- **Biopsy-confirmed MASH (the inflammatory form of fatty liver disease):** Particularly when fibrosis is present at stage 2 (some scar tissue bands present in the liver) or above. At this stage, the risk of progression to cirrhosis is meaningful, and the potential benefit of approved disease-modifying therapies is more clearly established.
- **Inadequate response to sustained lifestyle intervention:** People who have genuinely and consistently pursued dietary change, exercise, and weight loss for six to twelve months without adequate improvement in liver markers or disease stage may benefit from adjunctive pharmaceutical support.
- **Significant comorbidities:** People with type 2 diabetes, obesity, or cardiovascular disease often require pharmaceutical management of those conditions independently. Some of those medications—particularly GLP-1 agonists and SGLT2 inhibitors—have demonstrated

simultaneous liver benefits, making medication selection particularly relevant in this population.

- **Advanced or rapidly progressing disease:** In people with stage 3 to 4 fibrosis (significant scarring with impaired liver function; extensive scarring and severe liver damage) or cirrhosis, the therapeutic window for lifestyle-driven reversal narrows, and the urgency for effective intervention increases. Medication plays a more central role in the management of advanced disease.

To put this in perspective: The majority of people diagnosed with MASLD—particularly those at the steatosis or early MASH stage without significant fibrosis—will not meet these criteria with a genuine lifestyle effort. Large prospective studies show that five to ten percent weight loss alone produces meaningful reductions in liver fat and inflammation in most people. The criteria above describe exceptions and advanced presentations, not the expected trajectory for someone who commits to the approach in this book.

None of this means that medication is inevitable for anyone reading this book. The majority of people with early-stage fatty liver disease who commit to meaningful lifestyle change will not require pharmaceutical intervention. But knowing what is available—and under what circumstances it becomes relevant—is part of being an informed participant in your own care.

GLP-1 Receptor Agonists: The Most Discussed Drugs in Metabolic Medicine

No class of medications has received more attention in metabolic disease management over the past several years than GLP-1 receptor agonists. Originally developed for type 2 diabetes, drugs like semaglutide (Ozempic, Wegovy) and liraglutide (Saxenda, Victoza) have become household names through their dramatic weight loss effects—and their documented benefits for fatty liver disease have followed logically from that weight loss.

GLP-1 stands for glucagon-like peptide-1, a hormone naturally produced in the gut in response to food intake. It stimulates insulin secretion, suppresses glucagon (which drives blood sugar up), slows gastric emptying (making you feel full longer), and signals the brain's satiety centers to reduce appetite. Under normal circumstances, however, naturally produced GLP-1 is extraordinarily short-lived—it is broken down by an enzyme called DPP-4 within two to three minutes of release, meaning its effects are brief and tightly coupled to the moment of eating. GLP-1 receptor agonists are engineered analogs that mimic the hormone's actions while resisting that rapid breakdown—depending on the specific drug, they remain active for hours to a full week from a single injection. This prolonged biological presence is what distinguishes them pharmacologically from the body's own GLP-1 signal: rather than a brief pulse of appetite suppression tied to a meal, the drug delivers a sustained hormonal message that continuously reduces appetite, slows gastric emptying, and modulates blood sugar around the clock. The result is a degree of appetite suppression and metabolic effect that most people cannot achieve through willpower—or through any natural physiological process—alone.

What They Do for the Liver

The liver benefits of GLP-1 agonists in MASLD are documented and meaningful. Large clinical trials of semaglutide in people with MASH showed significant reductions in liver fat, improvements in liver inflammation, normalization of liver enzymes, and—in a proportion of participants—resolution of MASH on biopsy.[315] The ESSENCE trial, published in the *New England Journal of Medicine*, demonstrated that once-weekly semaglutide produced histological resolution of MASH without worsening fibrosis in approximately 63 percent of participants, compared to 34 percent of those receiving placebo.[316]

The mechanisms extend beyond weight loss. GLP-1 receptors are expressed in the liver, and direct receptor activation reduces *de novo* lipogenesis, improves hepatic insulin sensitivity, and decreases liver inflammation through pathways partially independent of body weight change.[317] GLP-1 agonists also reduce visceral fat preferentially—the metabolically active fat depot most directly implicated in driving liver inflammation—and improve cardiovascular risk markers that frequently accompany MASLD.[318]

The Risk Profile: What the Enthusiasm Sometimes Omits

GLP-1 agonists are potent medications with a real and significant side effect profile that deserves honest, complete disclosure—particularly given the pace at which they have entered popular culture as near-universal weight loss solutions.

- **Gastrointestinal effects:** Nausea, vomiting, diarrhea, and constipation are the most common adverse effects and affect a substantial proportion of users, particularly during dose escalation. For most people these effects are dose-dependent and improve over time, but a meaningful minority discontinue treatment because of them.

- **Gastroparesis (stomach paralysis):** GLP-1 agonists slow gastric motility as part of their mechanism. In some people, this progresses to clinically significant gastroparesis—a condition in which the stomach empties abnormally slowly, causing chronic nausea, vomiting, bloating, and pain. Cases of severe drug-induced gastroparesis requiring hospitalization have been reported with increasing frequency as GLP-1 agonist prescribing has expanded. People with pre-existing gastrointestinal motility disorders are at particular risk.
- **Pancreatitis:** An increased risk of acute pancreatitis has been observed in clinical trials and post-marketing surveillance. The absolute risk is low, but pancreatitis is a serious and potentially life-threatening condition, and people with a history of pancreatitis or gallbladder disease should discuss this risk carefully with their physician before starting GLP-1 therapy.
- **Gallbladder disease:** Rapid weight loss of any cause—and GLP-1 agonists can produce rapid weight loss—increases the risk of gallstone formation through the same bile concentration mechanism discussed in Chapter 6. Cholecystitis (gallbladder inflammation caused by gallstones) and cholelithiasis (gallstones in the gallbladder) are meaningfully more common in GLP-1 agonist users than in placebo groups in clinical trials.
- **Acute kidney injury:** Cases of acute kidney injury have been reported, likely related to dehydration from nausea and vomiting combined with reduced fluid intake. People with pre-existing kidney disease should be monitored closely.

- **Bone density:** Emerging data suggests that some of the weight lost with GLP-1 agonists comes from lean mass and bone mineral density rather than purely from fat tissue—a concern not relevant to lifestyle-based weight loss, where resistance training preserves muscle and bone. Essentially, the drug signals your brain that you're starving, so the body breaks down both fat and muscle to survive. This is an active area of investigation, but it reinforces the importance of maintaining resistance training during any weight loss program, pharmacologically assisted or otherwise.
- **Worsening diabetic retinopathy:** A paradoxical early worsening of diabetic eye disease was observed in some trial participants with pre-existing retinopathy. The mechanism is not fully understood but may relate to the rapid improvement in blood sugar control, which can temporarily stress retinal blood vessels. People with diabetic retinopathy should discuss this risk with their endocrinologist or ophthalmologist.
- **Nonarteritic anterior ischemic optic neuropathy (NAION):** A rare but serious form of optic nerve damage resulting in sudden vision loss has been reported in GLP-1 agonist users in several observational studies. The absolute risk appears low, but the severity of the outcome warrants attention, particularly for people with cardiovascular risk factors associated with NAION.
- **Mood changes:** Reports of depression, anxiety, suicidal ideation, and other mood changes in GLP-1 agonist users have prompted regulatory review in multiple countries. The causal relationship is not definitively established—obesity

and metabolic disease themselves carry elevated rates of depression—but the signal is sufficient to warrant monitoring, particularly in people with a psychiatric history.

- **Thyroid C-cell tumors:** GLP-1 receptor agonists carry a black box warning for thyroid C-cell tumors based on animal studies showing dose-dependent development of medullary thyroid carcinoma in rodents. Whether this risk translates to humans at clinical doses is not conclusively established, but GLP-1 agonists are contraindicated in people with a personal or family history of medullary thyroid carcinoma or multiple endocrine neoplasia syndrome type 2.
- **Weight regain upon discontinuation:** GLP-1 agonists suppress appetite through an externally supplied hormonal signal. When the medication is stopped, that signal disappears, appetite returns—often fully—and the majority of lost weight is typically regained within twelve to twenty-four months without sustained lifestyle change. This is not a moral failing; it is the pharmacology. It underscores why GLP-1 therapy is most appropriately viewed as a bridge or a catalyst, not a permanent solution that operates independently of lifestyle.

> **The Critical Framing.** *GLP-1 agonists are powerful and, for appropriate candidates, genuinely useful tools. They are not magic, and they are not without meaningful risk. The person best positioned to benefit from a GLP-1 agonist is one who uses it as a catalyst to establish lifestyle habits that can sustain the metabolic improvements after the medication is eventually reduced or stopped—not one who uses it as a substitute*

> *for those habits. Used that way, the medication and the lifestyle reinforce each other. Used as a standalone solution, the benefits are largely borrowed against a future bill that comes due when the prescription ends.*

It is also worth naming what GLP-1 medications cannot do: They do not repair the gut microbiome, reverse the circadian disruption underlying nighttime insulin dysfunction, reduce environmental toxin burden, or address the chronic stress physiology that contributes to fat deposition. They are a powerful, though risky, lever on appetite and weight—and a meaningful one for appropriate candidates—but the root-cause work described in this book is complementary and, for most people, comes first.

If You Choose to Use a GLP-1 or Similar Medication: A Practical Support Protocol

GLP-1 receptor agonists, tirzepatide, and agents like retatrutide (more to come on tirzepatide and retatrutide) are powerful metabolic tools—but their potency creates specific physiological demands that require deliberate management. Appetite suppression this significant, and weight loss this rapid, does not come without trade-offs. The following protocol is designed to protect what matters most while the medication does its work.

Protect Your Muscle First

This is not optional. The most consequential risk of aggressive pharmacologically assisted weight loss is the loss of lean muscle tissue alongside fat—a trade-off that undermines long-term metabolic health and is largely avoidable with the right approach.

These medications work, in part, by significantly reducing how much you eat. That sounds straightforwardly good—and for many people, it is. But your body does not distinguish neatly between fat and muscle when it begins drawing down its energy reserves. Eat considerably less without a deliberate strategy to protect lean tissue, and a meaningful portion of the weight you lose will come from muscle. For someone with MASLD, that is a serious problem.

Here is why it matters: Muscle is metabolically active tissue. It is one of the primary sites where your body disposes of blood sugar and improves insulin sensitivity. Losing it undermines the very mechanism you are trying to restore. You may weigh less on the scale while becoming more metabolically fragile—a trade most people would not knowingly accept.

This is a reason to use GLP-1 medications smarter if they are appropriate for you.

Target protein intake of 0.7 to 1 gram per pound of body weight daily, distributed across meals rather than concentrated in one sitting. Prioritize leucine-rich protein sources—whey protein, Greek yogurt, cottage cheese, eggs, and lean meats—because leucine is the primary trigger for muscle protein synthesis through the mTOR pathway. When appetite is significantly suppressed, getting adequate protein becomes harder than it sounds; treat it as a non-negotiable nutritional priority, ahead of carbohydrates and fats, at every meal.

Resistance training three to five times per week is equally non-negotiable. Focus on compound movements—squats, deadlifts, rows, presses—that recruit the largest muscle groups and provide the strongest retention signal. Apply progressive overload: Even modest attempts to maintain or increase the weight lifted while in a caloric deficit preserve the muscle stimulus that medication alone cannot provide.

When lifestyle changes, adequate protein intake, and targeted supplementation are layered intentionally alongside a GLP-1 agonist, the picture changes substantially. Three evidence-informed tools—creatine, HMB, and fortetropin—each address a different piece of the muscle-preservation puzzle, and they work well together.

Creatine monohydrate (5 grams daily) is among the most studied and well-supported sports science supplements in existence, with a safety and efficacy record spanning decades.[319] It works by replenishing phosphocreatine in muscle tissue, which fuels short, high-intensity muscular contractions—resistance training, primarily. During a caloric deficit (which GLP-1 medications reliably create), creatine helps sustain training performance and supports muscle cell hydration and volume, both of which signal the body to preserve lean tissue rather than cannibalize it. The standard dose is straightforward: five grams daily, no loading phase required for most people. It is inexpensive, well-tolerated, and deserves to be a default—not an afterthought—for anyone on a GLP-1 who is also doing resistance training.

HMB (beta-hydroxy beta-methylbutyrate), is a metabolite of leucine, the amino acid most responsible for triggering muscle protein synthesis. HMB's primary role is anti-catabolic: It slows the rate at which muscle protein breaks down, which matters enormously during periods of reduced caloric intake. Clinical research has consistently shown that HMB supplementation offsets muscle loss during caloric restriction—which is precisely the metabolic environment a GLP-1 agonist creates.[320] A typical effective dose is one to three grams daily, with the free acid form (HMB-FA) showing faster absorption than the calcium salt form (HMB-Ca). For someone who is older, less physically active, or who has already lost muscle mass through prior weight cycling, HMB may be especially valuable.

Fortetropin is the newest and most targeted of the three. It is a naturally derived myofibrillar protein concentrate extracted from fertilized egg yolk that has been specifically studied for its effect on muscle protein synthesis—not just preservation, but active anabolic signaling.[321] Six clinical trials have examined fortetropin's effects, including in older adults and individuals in calorie-restricted states.[322] Across these studies, fortetropin has demonstrated a meaningful ability to increase lean muscle mass and reduce muscle protein breakdown (by inhibiting myostatin—a protein that limits muscle growth), with effects appearing to occur through pathways that support muscle growth even in conditions where building new muscle is physiologically difficult—such as during significant caloric restriction or aging-related anabolic resistance.

At the cellular level, fortetropin flips the biological "switch" relatively quickly. In some studies, the initial myostatin-lowering effects begins within 72 hours, although it may not be measurable in serum. The key milestone in human research is 21 days. After 21 days of consistent supplementation, the rate of muscle protein synthesis increased by 18 percent, suggesting the body has shifted into a more anabolic state. Functional and mobility improvements follow at 4 to 8 weeks, while measurable muscle mass and body composition changes require 12 weeks and beyond.

Even more importantly, fortetropin has been evaluated alongside GLP-1 therapy in a preclinical trial.[323] The obese animal model demonstrated that fortetropin preserves muscle mass and supports metabolic health during weight loss with a low-caloric diet or induced by GLP-1 receptor agonists. Specifically, fortetropin supplementation preserved calf muscle mass and improved glucose tolerance compared to the control group. This research suggests fortetropin is a promising strategy for maintaining muscle mass, strength, and metabolic health during medical weight loss.

This is what makes fortetropin particularly relevant in the context of GLP-1 therapy. Creatine supports training performance. HMB slows breakdown. Fortetropin actively supports the rebuilding signal. Together, they create a layered defense around the muscle tissue you already have, while giving your body the biological inputs it needs to respond to resistance exercise and rebuild rather than simply lose less.

Vitamin D and omega-3 fatty acids—already discussed in Chapter 9—support muscle fiber contraction, strength, and the muscle protein synthetic response to amino acids. If you are already taking these for liver health, continue them. If you are not, a GLP-1 protocol is a strong additional reason to start.

If you are on or considering a GLP-1 agonist, here is a practical framework to protect your muscle throughout treatment:

- **Prioritize protein**. Aim for 1.2 to 1.6 grams of protein per kilogram of body weight daily, distributed across meals. On a GLP-1, appetite suppression can make this feel difficult—make protein the first priority at each meal, not the last.
- **Resistance train consistently**. Two to three sessions per week is enough. This is non-negotiable. Without a stimulus to

preserve and rebuild muscle, no supplement will fully compensate.

- **Add creatine monohydrate**. Five grams daily with food. Long-term use is safe and supported by extensive research.
- **Consider HMB**. One to three grams daily, particularly during periods of rapid weight loss or if resistance training is limited.
- **Consider fortetropin**. The clinically studied dose used in trials is approximately 6.6 grams daily (best taken after exercise and mixed in a smoothie). It pairs naturally with creatine and HMB as part of a complete muscle-support strategy, not as a replacement for any one of them.
- **Begin or continue vitamin D and omega-3 fatty acids supplementation**. These two supplements support muscle health.

These are not magic. No supplement is. But they represent the strongest evidence-based tools currently available for preserving metabolic tissue during medically assisted weight loss—and that distinction matters far more than most people realize.

Support Your Digestive System

Because these medications significantly slow gastric emptying, the gut needs deliberate support. Constipation is common; so is the distinctive gastric discomfort sometimes described as sulfur burps, caused by food sitting in the stomach longer than usual.

Maintain fiber intake at 25 to 35 grams per day—but increase gradually if your current intake is low. A sudden jump in fiber while gastric motility is slowed amplifies bloating and discomfort rather than relieving it. Add one high-fiber food at a time and give the system several days to adjust before adding another.

Hydration requires active attention. These medications can blunt thirst signals, increasing the risk of dehydration that compounds nausea and can contribute to the kidney stress noted in earlier. Prioritize consistent water intake throughout the day rather than waiting for thirst. An electrolyte supplement containing magnesium and potassium supports both hydration and muscle function—particularly important if nausea is reducing your overall food and fluid intake.

Some people find that digestive enzyme supplements containing lipase or protease reduce the heaviness and fullness associated with slower gastric emptying. This is a reasonable and low-risk addition if gastrointestinal comfort is a limiting factor in tolerability. Take these before meals.

Protect Gallbladder and Metabolic Function

As discussed in the side effect section, rapid weight loss meaningfully increases gallstone risk. Include small amounts of healthy fat—olive oil, avocado, nuts—at each meal to stimulate gallbladder contraction and bile flow. Staying well hydrated further reduces bile concentration. This is not a guarantee against gallstone formation, but it meaningfully reduces the risk.

Even if you are not using the medication for diabetes, GLP-1 drugs affect insulin sensitivity in ways that can occasionally cause low blood sugar—particularly when combined with intense exercise. Be aware of the symptoms of hypoglycemia (dizziness, shakiness, sudden fatigue) and discuss monitoring with your prescribing physician if you are exercising vigorously.

Prioritize Micronutrient Density

When total food volume drops significantly, the risk of subclinical micronutrient deficiencies rises quietly. With less food comes less opportunity for the vitamins, minerals, and trace elements that support liver function, immune health, hormonal balance, and energy metabolism. Every meal should prioritize nutrient density over caloric volume: vegetables, quality proteins, legumes, and healthy fats rather than filling the reduced appetite with nutritionally thin foods. A comprehensive multinutrient supplement is a reasonable insurance policy during this period.

Address Skin, Hair, and Connective Tissue

Rapid fat loss can outpace the skin's ability to adapt, and significant caloric restriction can trigger temporary hair shedding—a condition called telogen effluvium—typically appearing two to four months after the period of rapid weight loss. Both are largely manageable.

Collagen peptides at 10 to 20 grams daily provide the specific amino acids—hydroxyproline and proline—that support skin elasticity and joint integrity during periods of rapid body composition change. Biotin and zinc support the keratin infrastructure of hair and nails, which can become brittle during periods of significant metabolic flux. Neither is a guarantee, but both are low-risk, low-cost additions with relevant biological rationale.

Sleep Remains the Foundation

The metabolic shifts driven by these medications can sometimes interfere with sleep architecture. Simultaneously, sleep deprivation elevates cortisol—which directly counteracts both the muscle-sparing and fat-loss effects of the medication, as established in Chapter 7.

Seven to nine hours of quality sleep per night is not a lifestyle preference while on these medications. It is a clinical priority that determines in part how effectively the drug is working.

Pioglitazone: The Established Option for Diabetic Patients

Pioglitazone is a thiazolidinedione—a class of medication that improves insulin sensitivity by activating PPAR-gamma receptors in fat tissue, muscle, and the liver. It has been used for type 2 diabetes management for over two decades and has one of the more consistent evidence bases for MASH of any pharmacological agent,[324] predating the newer generation of metabolic drugs by many years.

In clinical trials of people with biopsy-confirmed MASH, pioglitazone has consistently produced significant improvements in liver fat, liver inflammation, ballooning degeneration of liver cells, and fibrosis.[325] A major meta-analysis of pioglitazone trials found that it produced histological improvement in MASH in approximately 50 percent of participants—meaningful, though lower than the resolution rates seen with semaglutide in more recent trials.[326] It also reduces fasting glucose, triglycerides, and ALT levels and has cardiovascular benefit data in people with type 2 diabetes.

The primary benefits-risk considerations with pioglitazone:

- **Weight gain:** Pioglitazone consistently causes weight gain—typically two to four kilograms—primarily through fluid retention and an increase in subcutaneous (not visceral) fat. This weight gain is metabolically different from the harmful visceral fat accumulation that drives liver disease, but it is nonetheless a common concern for people who are managing obesity.

- **Fluid retention and heart failure risk:** Pioglitazone promotes sodium and water retention, which can worsen or precipitate heart failure in susceptible individuals. It is contraindicated in people with existing heart failure.
- **Bone fracture risk:** Long-term pioglitazone use is associated with increased fracture risk, particularly in women, due to effects on bone metabolism. This is a relevant consideration for people already at elevated fracture risk.
- **Potential bladder cancer association:** Some epidemiological data has suggested a modest increased risk of bladder cancer with long-term pioglitazone use, though the evidence is not conclusive and the absolute risk is low. Regulatory agencies have not withdrawn the medication but recommend caution in people with a history of bladder cancer.

Current guidelines consider pioglitazone primarily for people with MASH who also have type 2 diabetes, in whom the dual metabolic and hepatic benefits are most clearly established. In nondiabetic MASH, the evidence is also supportive, but the benefit-risk calculation requires more individualized assessment. It is an older, less expensive medication with a well-characterized safety profile—an important practical consideration in discussions of treatment access and affordability.

Resmetirom: The First FDA-Approved Drug Specifically for MASH

In March 2024, the FDA approved resmetirom (brand name Rezdiffra) for the treatment of adults with noncirrhotic MASH with moderate to advanced fibrosis—making it the first drug specifically approved for MASH rather than for a comorbidity that happens to benefit the liver. This is a genuinely significant milestone in the history of fatty liver disease treatment, and it warrants explanation of what it actually does and what it means in practice.

Resmetirom is a selective thyroid hormone receptor beta (THR-beta) agonist. To understand why that matters, a brief analogy helps: thyroid hormone has two main receptors. THR-alpha is distributed widely in the heart, bone, and brain, and stimulating it produces the side effects associated with hyperthyroidism—racing heart, bone loss, anxiety. THR-beta is concentrated heavily in the liver and is the receptor responsible for thyroid hormone's effects on fat metabolism, cholesterol processing, and mitochondrial function in hepatic tissue. Resmetirom selectively activates THR-beta while largely sparing THR-alpha, delivering the liver-specific metabolic benefits of thyroid hormone activity without the systemic side effects of a hyperthyroid state.

What the Trial Data Shows

The MAESTRO-NASH trial, the pivotal study leading to FDA approval, enrolled over 900 adults with biopsy-confirmed MASH with fibrosis stage 2 or 3.[327] At the primary endpoints—MASH resolution without worsening fibrosis, and fibrosis improvement by at least one stage—resmetirom at 100 mg daily significantly outperformed placebo. Approximately 26 percent of resmetirom-treated participants achieved MASH resolution (versus 10 percent on a placebo), and approximately 24 percent showed fibrosis improvement (versus 14 percent on a placebo).

The drug also produced significant reductions in liver fat (measured by MRI), improvements in liver enzymes, and favorable shifts in lipid and metabolic markers. Secondary analyses suggested additional cardiovascular benefit through LDL cholesterol reduction and non-HDL cholesterol improvements.

These are meaningful results—genuine, statistically significant, histologically confirmed improvements in a serious liver disease. They are also, it is worth noting, far from complete responses. Roughly three-quarters of treated participants did not achieve MASH resolution or fibrosis improvement by the primary endpoints. Resmetirom is an advance, not a cure, and the majority of people taking it will still require ongoing lifestyle management to achieve and maintain the best possible outcomes.

Side Effects and Practical Considerations

The most common adverse effects of resmetirom are gastrointestinal—nausea and diarrhea, most pronounced during the early weeks of treatment and generally diminishing over time. Pruritus (itching) has been reported in some participants. Liver enzyme elevations occurred in a small proportion of treated patients and resolved upon dose reduction or discontinuation.

Resmetirom carries a risk of drug interactions through CYP2C8 and CYP3A4 enzyme pathways, which are relevant for people taking other medications metabolized by these enzymes. It is not approved for people with decompensated cirrhosis and requires monitoring of liver function during treatment.

Cost and access are practical realities worth acknowledging: As a newly approved branded medication for a specific indication, resmetirom is expensive, and insurance coverage varies. The conversation with your prescribing physician should include a realistic assessment of access, coverage, and the monitoring requirements that come with the medication.

Resmetirom represents the leading edge of a new era in MASH pharmacotherapy. It is the most disease-specific option currently approved, it has a plausible and well-characterized mechanism, and it has demonstrated genuine histological benefit in a rigorously conducted trial. For people with moderate to advanced fibrosis who have not achieved adequate improvement through lifestyle intervention alone, it is a meaningful option to discuss with a hepatologist.

SGLT2 Inhibitors: Cardiovascular Drugs with Liver Benefits

SGLT2 inhibitors—including empagliflozin (Jardiance), dapagliflozin (Farxiga), and canagliflozin (Invokana)—are a class of diabetes medications that work by blocking sodium-glucose cotransporter 2 in the kidneys, preventing reabsorption of filtered glucose and causing it to be excreted in the urine. The result is a glucose-lowering effect that operates independently of insulin, along with meaningful weight loss, blood pressure reduction, and—documented in landmark cardiovascular trials—substantial reductions in heart failure hospitalizations and cardiovascular mortality in high-risk patients.[328,329]

Their relevance to fatty liver disease emerged from secondary analyses of these cardiovascular trials and from dedicated MASLD studies. SGLT2 inhibitors consistently reduce liver fat, lower liver enzymes, and improve markers of insulin resistance in people with MASLD who also have type 2 diabetes. A number of smaller trials in nondiabetic MASLD populations have shown similar signals, though the evidence base is less mature than for the diabetic population.[330]

The mechanisms are several: Caloric loss through glycosuria (glucose excreted in urine represents lost calories), reduction in plasma insulin levels, visceral fat reduction, and direct effects on hepatic fat metabolism that appear partially independent of weight loss.

The side effect profile of SGLT2 inhibitors is generally favorable compared to some other metabolic medications:

- **Genital mycotic infections:** The most common adverse effect—increased glucose in the urine creates a favorable environment for yeast infections in both men and women. Usually mild and manageable.
- **Urinary tract infections:** Modestly increased risk, related to the same glucosuric mechanism.
- **Diabetic ketoacidosis:** A rare but serious complication, including cases occurring at normal blood glucose levels (euglycemic DKA), which can delay diagnosis. Risk is higher during illness, surgery, or significant dietary restriction.
- **Volume depletion:** The osmotic diuresis effect can cause dehydration, particularly in the elderly or those taking diuretics. Blood pressure lowering can be excessive in some individuals.
- **Lower limb amputation risk:** Canagliflozin specifically has carried an FDA warning for increased risk of lower limb amputation, particularly the toes, observed in clinical trials. This risk appears to be lower with other agents in the class and is higher among people with poorly controlled diabetes and pre-existing heart of blood vessel problems.

SGLT2 inhibitors are not currently FDA-approved specifically for MASLD—their liver benefits are documented but the indication has not been formally pursued for this disease. In clinical practice, they are primarily relevant for people with MASLD who also have type 2 diabetes or established cardiovascular disease, in whom the cardiometabolic benefits are independently indicated and the liver improvements are a meaningful additional gain.

Off-Label and Adjunctive Approaches

Beyond the primary agents discussed above, several medications are used off-label or in adjunctive roles in the management of fatty liver disease and its metabolic drivers. These are not formally approved for MASLD but have evidence-based rationale in appropriate clinical contexts.

Metformin

Metformin is the world's most prescribed diabetes medication and shares its primary mechanism—AMPK activation—with the supplement berberine discussed in Chapter 9. Despite strong theoretical rationale and favorable metabolic effects, metformin has not shown consistent benefit for liver histology in MASH clinical trials.[331,332] It improves insulin sensitivity and metabolic markers, but multiple dedicated MASH trials have not demonstrated meaningful improvements in liver fat, inflammation, or fibrosis compared to placebos. Current guidelines do not recommend metformin specifically for MASH management.

However, metformin is often appropriate for people with MASLD who have prediabetes or type 2 diabetes—not for its liver-specific effects, but for its well-established glycemic benefits and its favorable safety and cost profile. In that context, it is a reasonable component of a comprehensive metabolic management plan even though it is not a primary liver therapy.

Statins

Statins are often avoided by people with liver disease—and by some clinicians managing it—out of concern that these cholesterol-lowering drugs might further stress a liver that is already compromised. This concern, while understandable, is largely unsupported by the evidence and has led to undertreatment of cardiovascular risk in a population that is at significantly elevated cardiovascular risk.

The evidence actually suggests that statins are safe in the majority of people with MASLD and may be modestly hepatoprotective—associated in some studies with lower rates of liver enzyme elevation, reduced hepatic inflammation, and possibly lower progression rates.[333] They are primarily indicated for people with MASLD who have elevated cardiovascular risk, elevated LDL cholesterol, or established cardiovascular disease, and the fear of statin hepatotoxicity should not prevent their use in appropriately selected patients.

True statin-induced hepatotoxicity is rare—estimated at approximately one in 100,000 users. The mild transaminase elevations that occur in a small proportion of statin users are typically not clinically significant and do not reflect genuine liver injury. The common practice of avoiding statins in anyone with elevated liver enzymes—without distinguishing between MASLD-related elevation and drug-induced injury—is not supported by current hepatology guidelines and deprives a high-risk population of meaningful cardiovascular protection.

If you have been advised to avoid statins because of your fatty liver disease and you have elevated cardiovascular risk, this is a conversation worth having explicitly with both your cardiologist and your hepatologist. The risk-benefit calculation is, for some people with MASLD, favorable toward statin use, but many integrative-minded cardiologists are reducing their use altogether.

Statins come with some notable potential side effects that doctors and patients should discuss. One common issue is muscle pain (myalgia) or weakness, which can range from mild discomfort to, in rare cases, more serious muscle damage. Many experts believe this may be linked to depletion of CoQ10, a natural substance in the body that helps produce energy in cells—some people take CoQ10 supplements to try to ease these symptoms, though evidence on its effectiveness is mixed. It may also have to do with inhibition of heme A by statins, which disrupts the electron transport chain, reducing cellular energy efficiency and accelerating mitochondrial dysfunction.

An emerging risk is brain disorders. Statins deplete dolichol—a vital molecule concentrated in the substantia nigra (a brain region linked to movement control. Lower dolichol levels may increase the risk of Parkinson's disease and other neurodegenerative disorders. Since your brain is predominantly fat, unnaturally reducing cholesterol may contribute to poor cognitive function and memory problems, especially in older adults.

Statins interfere with the liver's production of cholesterol—where 80 percent of your cholesterol comes from. Indeed, they reduce cholesterol synthesis too much. Artificially suppressing cholesterol production may lead to hormonal imbalances, reduced vitamin D synthesis, diminished cell membrane integrity, cognitive decline, and even mental health issues.

Lastly, statins don't actually address the root cause of heart disease, which is chronic inflammation, insulin resistance, oxidative stress, and poor diet and lifestyle. Instead of simply lowering cholesterol, lifestyle and dietary interventions, combined with targeted nutraceuticals should be first line treatment options.

Other frequent complaints include digestive problems like nausea, constipation, diarrhea, or stomach upset. Statins can also cause a modest rise in blood sugar levels, which over time may increase the risk of developing type 2 diabetes in certain individuals, particularly those already at higher risk.

While most people tolerate statins well and serious complications are uncommon, these side effects are why regular check-ins with your doctor are important—they can often adjust the dose, switch medications, or monitor you closely to balance the heart-protective benefits against the downsides. Always talk to your healthcare provider before starting or stopping statins.

Vitamin E (Pharmaceutical Context)

Vitamin E at 800 IU per day—discussed in Chapter 9 in the supplement context—meets the threshold for a meaningful pharmacological intervention in its specific indicated population: nondiabetic adults with biopsy-confirmed MASH. The PIVENS trial's findings position it as a legitimate option in this narrow but real group, and it is referenced in AASLD guidelines accordingly.[334] In people with MASLD who are diabetic, have cardiovascular disease, or are at elevated risk for prostate cancer, the risk-benefit calculation is less clearly favorable, and the decision should be made with a physician.

One safety consideration deserves specific attention, particularly for men. The large SELECT trial—which enrolled over 35,000 healthy men—found that those taking 400 IU of isolated alpha-tocopherol daily had an approximately 17 percent higher relative risk of prostate cancer compared to a placebo over roughly seven years, translating to about eleven additional cases per thousand men. Understanding why this happens clarifies how to use vitamin E intelligently rather than simply avoiding it.

Most standard vitamin E supplements contain only alpha-tocopherol—one of eight naturally occurring forms of vitamin E. At high supplemental doses, alpha-tocopherol competes with and actively depletes gamma-tocopherol in blood and tissues. This matters because gamma-tocopherol has distinct anti-inflammatory and anti-proliferative properties that alpha-tocopherol lacks, and it appears to be protective against prostate cancer specifically. Flooding the system with isolated alpha-tocopherol disrupts the natural balance of tocopherol forms—a balance that food sources of vitamin E, including nuts, seeds, and vegetable oils, preserve naturally.

High-dose isolated alpha-tocopherol can also behave as a pro-oxidant rather than an antioxidant in certain cellular contexts, potentially increasing oxidative stress in prostate tissue rather than reducing it. The practical solution is not to abandon vitamin E supplementation where it is clinically indicated, but to use mixed tocopherol formulations—products that include gamma-tocopherol, delta-tocopherol, and other naturally occurring forms alongside alpha—which preserve the biological balance found in whole foods and avoid the gamma-tocopherol displacement that appears to drive the prostate cancer signal.

Men with prostate cancer risk factors, and anyone taking high-dose vitamin E for an extended period, should discuss the specific form and dose with their physician before proceeding. The natural d-alpha form is preferable to the synthetic dl-alpha form under any circumstances, but mixed tocopherols are the more complete and safer choice for long-term supplemental use.

The Pipeline: What Is Coming

The MASLD pharmaceutical pipeline is the most active it has ever been—a reflection of both the urgency of the global epidemic and the gaps that lifestyle intervention alone cannot close in the most advanced cases of disease. For people with stage 3–4 fibrosis or cirrhosis, where the window for lifestyle-driven reversal has narrowed significantly, this pipeline matters enormously. For the majority of readers of this book—those in earlier disease stages with significant reversibility—it is background knowledge more than actionable guidance. Understanding where pharmacology is heading helps contextualize the landscape, but the most durable investment remains the one that works regardless of what gets approved: the foundation you are building now.

FXR agonists (farnesoid X receptor): Bile acid receptor agonists that modulate hepatic fat metabolism, inflammation, and fibrosis. Obeticholic acid showed meaningful fibrosis improvement in the REGENERATE trial but was not approved due to an unfavorable benefit-risk profile at that time;[335] next-generation FXR agonists with improved tolerability are in development.

Dual and triple hormone receptor agonists: This is arguably the most closely watched space in all of metabolic medicine. Tirzepatide (Mounjaro, Zepbound), already approved for type 2 diabetes and obesity, combines GLP-1 and GIP receptor agonism and has shown highly promising early MASLD signals in Phase 2 trials, with MASH resolution rates exceeding those seen with semaglutide alone.[336]

To understand why tirzepatide and its successors represent a meaningful pharmacological advance rather than simply "more of the same," it helps to understand what the GIP receptor adds—and why its inclusion changes the character of the drug in ways that go beyond incremental potency.

GIP stands for glucose-dependent insulinotropic polypeptide, a hormone released from the upper small intestine in response to fat and carbohydrate ingestion.[337] Like GLP-1, it stimulates insulin secretion in a glucose-dependent manner. But GIP has a distinct and important additional role: It acts on adipose tissue directly, promoting fat storage when calories are abundant and—critically—fat mobilization and oxidation when the body is in an energy deficit. GIP receptor signaling also appears to modulate dopamine pathways in the brain differently from GLP-1, producing a subtly different appetite and reward signal that may explain why the combination produces greater weight loss than either hormone alone.[338] Perhaps most relevant to tolerability: GIP receptor agonism appears to counteract some of the gastrointestinal side effects associated with pure GLP-1 receptor activation. GLP-1 receptor agonism alone slows gastric motility and triggers nausea through vagal nerve pathways; GIP receptor co-activation appears to modulate this effect, which is one proposed mechanism for why tirzepatide produces less nausea and vomiting per unit of weight loss than semaglutide at comparable doses. Think of it this way: GLP-1 agonism applies the brake on appetite and gastric emptying firmly and somewhat bluntly, while GIP co-agonism helps modulate that brake—producing a smoother, better-tolerated deceleration toward the same metabolic destination.

The clinical trial evidence bears this out. In the SURMOUNT trials of tirzepatide for obesity, gastrointestinal adverse events—nausea, vomiting, and diarrhea—occurred at rates broadly comparable to or modestly lower than those seen with semaglutide in the STEP trials, despite tirzepatide producing greater overall weight loss.[339] Discontinuation rates due to adverse events were also somewhat lower for tirzepatide in head-to-head analyses, suggesting that the dual mechanism improves tolerability without sacrificing efficacy. Importantly, some researchers report that tirzepatide shows a more favorable muscle mass preservation profile than GLP-1 agonists alone in some analyses—possibly because GIP receptor signaling on adipose tissue improves the specificity of fat mobilization, reducing the proportion of weight lost that comes from lean tissue.[340] This is a meaningful advantage given the muscle loss concern raised throughout this chapter, though it does not eliminate the need for resistance training and adequate protein—it simply makes the ceiling on muscle preservation somewhat higher. However, because Tirzepatide is so incredibly powerful at helping you lose weight, it can be a double-edged sword. If you lose weight too quickly without eating enough protein or lifting weights, you might actually lose more muscle than you would on a weaker drug. The "favorable profile" only works if you give your body the protein and exercise it needs to keep that muscle strong.

Retatrutide, currently in Phase 3 trials under Eli Lilly's TRIUMPH program, goes a step further—targeting GLP-1, GIP, and glucagon receptors simultaneously, making it the first triple hormone receptor agonist to reach this stage of development. Phase 2 data published in the *New England Journal of Medicine* showed 24.2 percent weight loss at 48 weeks,[341] and Phase 3 TRIUMPH-4 data reported in December 2025 extended that to 28.7 percent at 68 weeks—the highest weight loss ever recorded in a randomized controlled trial of any obesity medication.[342] A dedicated Phase 2a trial of retatrutide specifically in MASLD, published in *Nature Medicine*, documented significant reductions in liver fat and improvements in metabolic markers,[343] establishing its relevance for fatty liver disease specifically and not just obesity broadly. Regulatory approval is not expected before 2027 at the earliest, as Eli Lilly had not yet filed a New Drug Application as of mid-2026.

A significant caution is worth naming directly: Weight loss of this magnitude and pace—with some individuals losing weight considerably faster than a safe 1 to 2 pounds per week—carries the same risks described in Chapter 6 for aggressive weight loss: accelerated gallstone formation, temporary worsening of liver inflammation from rapid fatty acid mobilization, and substantial loss of lean muscle mass alongside fat. The clinical trials for retatrutide are beginning to grapple with these questions, and the dysesthesia signal—skin sensitivity and tingling affecting roughly one in five participants on higher doses—adds another layer of monitoring complexity. Extraordinary efficacy and extraordinary side effect potential tend to travel together. If retatrutide reaches approval and eventually becomes available for MASLD management, the principles in Chapter 6 and in the GLP-1 agonist section about protecting muscle through resistance training and adequate protein will be more important, not less, for people using it.

The pancreatic and gallbladder risks associated with GLP-1 agonists appear to persist with dual and triple agonists, as these risks are at least partly mediated through the GLP-1 receptor component that all agents in this class share. Similarly, the cardiovascular safety profile of tirzepatide, while favorable overall—with emerging data suggesting cardiovascular event reduction in high-risk populations—continues to be characterized in ongoing trials. The dysesthesia signal observed with retatrutide in Phase 3, affecting roughly one in five participants at higher doses, appears specific to the triple agonist mechanism and has not been reported with the same frequency for tirzepatide, suggesting that glucagon receptor co-agonism may introduce side effect dimensions that GLP-1 and GIP agonism alone do not. Glucagon receptor activation also raises theoretical concerns about hepatic glucose output and potential effects on bone density that require longer-term data to fully characterize. The bottom line on comparative safety: dual agonists appear to offer a meaningfully improved tolerability profile relative to pure GLP-1 agonists; triple agonists deliver greater efficacy still, but with an evolving and not yet fully characterized side effect landscape that warrants appropriate caution until longer-term post-marketing data accumulates.

MOTS-c: Here's a fascinating idea: what if your body already produces a molecule that mimics the metabolic effects of exercise—and what if people with MASLD have less of it?

That's not science fiction. It's the story of MOTS-c, and it's one of the more exciting developments in metabolic medicine right now.

MOTS-c (pronounced "motts-see") stands for Mitochondrial Open Reading Frame of the 12S rRNA-c. The name is a mouthful, so let's simplify it: MOTS-c is a tiny signaling peptide—just 16 amino acids long—that is encoded not by your regular DNA, but by the DNA inside your mitochondria. That's unusual and important. Your mitochondria are the energy-generating engines of your cells, and for decades, scientists assumed their DNA only handled the basics of energy production. MOTS-c changed that assumption entirely.

What researchers discovered is that MOTS-c functions more like a hormone than a structural protein. It is released in response to metabolic stress, travels through the bloodstream, enters cells—and even migrates into the cell nucleus—where it essentially flips on genes that restore metabolic balance. Think of it as your mitochondria sending an emergency signal that says: the energy system is under strain; let's fix it.

The reason MOTS-c has caught the attention of liver and metabolic researchers is what it does once it gets to work. MOTS-c plays its key physiological roles primarily through activating the AICAR-AMPK signaling pathway, which helps reduce insulin resistance, prevent obesity, and improve muscle function.[344] If AMPK sounds familiar, it should—it's the same energy-sensing switch that exercise activates. It's also the primary target of metformin, one of the most widely prescribed diabetes medications in the world.

In animal studies, MOTS-c treatment prevented both age-dependent and high-fat-diet-induced insulin resistance, as well as diet-induced obesity.[345] When researchers gave MOTS-c to mice fed a high-fat diet, it did not impact food intake—instead, it increased energy expenditure, as indicated by increased heat output. These mice had less fat accumulation due to increased carbohydrate usage and increased beta oxidation of fatty acids. In plain terms: the body burned more fat and stored less of it—including in the liver.

In MASLD and fibrosis models, MOTS-c has been shown to activate AMPK, regulate nuclear gene expression, suppress fibrotic and inflammatory signaling, and restore mitochondrial function.[346] That's a remarkable range of effects for a single molecule—and every one of those actions addresses a core driver of MASLD progression.

There's also an interesting human connection. In a cohort study, plasma MOTS-c levels in men were negatively correlated with fasting insulin levels, glycosylated hemoglobin, and body mass index.[347] In other words, the people with the worst metabolic markers tended to have the lowest levels of this protective peptide. That's a meaningful signal, even if it doesn't yet prove causation.

It's worth being candid here about the current state of MOTS-c science, because the enthusiasm surrounding it can outpace the evidence.

The bulk of what we know comes from animal studies and laboratory models. Human clinical trials with MOTS-c as a therapeutic peptide are ongoing. A modified analog of MOTS-c called CB4211 showed early promise in preclinical research—in cell culture, CB4211 enhanced insulin-mediated reduction of glucose in liver cells and inhibited lipolysis in fat cells—but its path through formal clinical trials is still unfolding.[348]

MOTS-c is increasingly recognized as an "exercise mimetic" peptide, and that framing captures both its promise and its current limitations. The idea of replicating the metabolic benefits of exercise in a molecule is genuinely exciting—especially for people who face physical limitations, advanced metabolic dysfunction, or simply need a therapeutic boost alongside lifestyle change. But "exercise mimetic" should not be read as "exercise replacement." The lifestyle foundations in this book remain your most powerful tools, precisely because they activate many of the same pathways MOTS-c influences—naturally, safely, and right now.

MOTS-c belongs in your awareness, not yet in your therapeutic repertoire. Peptide therapies are not regulated by the FDA in the same way pharmaceuticals are, quality and dosing standards are inconsistent, and long-term safety in humans is not yet established. Some clinics and compounding pharmacies offer MOTS-c injections as a wellness therapy, but these are well ahead of the clinical evidence.

What this research does tell you is something genuinely encouraging: your own body has metabolic repair systems built into its most fundamental machinery. Exercise, quality sleep, metabolic eating, and stress reduction all support the natural production of MOTS-c and the pathways it activates. You don't have to wait for a clinical trial to benefit from what the science behind MOTS-c is revealing. You're already working with the same system—every time you go for a walk, cut back on sugar, or get a full night's sleep.

Keep an eye on MOTS-c. The science is moving quickly, and if early findings hold up in human trials, it could become a meaningful tool in the metabolic medicine toolkit—particularly for people with advanced insulin resistance or MASH who need more than lifestyle changes alone.

FGF21 analogues (efruxifermin, pegozafermin, and others): Fibroblast growth factor 21 is sometimes described as the body's natural "metabolic stress hormone"—a signal released primarily by the liver during fasting, prolonged exercise, and states of nutrient deprivation that coordinates a shift toward fat burning, reduced lipid accumulation, and cellular protection across multiple organ systems simultaneously. The problem with natural FGF21 is the same problem that led to the development of GLP-1 agonists from natural GLP-1: It is broken down within minutes, making it pharmacologically useless in its native form. FGF21 analogues are engineered, long-acting versions of this hormone—modified to resist rapid degradation while preserving and amplifying the hormone's biological actions.

What makes FGF21 analogues particularly interesting for MASLD is the breadth of their mechanism. Unlike resmetirom, which works primarily in the liver through thyroid hormone receptor activation, FGF21 analogues act on multiple tissues simultaneously through FGFR1c and beta-Klotho receptors. In the liver, they suppress *de novo* lipogenesis, increase fatty acid oxidation, and reduce lipid influx—addressing fat accumulation from multiple directions at once. They also activate the Nrf2 antioxidant pathway and support autophagy (the cellular housekeeping process), protecting hepatocytes from the oxidative stress and lipotoxicity that drive the transition from steatosis to active hepatitis. Critically, they inhibit hepatic stellate cell activation—the fibrosis-generating machinery in the liver—producing anti-fibrotic effects that are not merely a downstream consequence of reduced inflammation but appear to operate through partially direct mechanisms. Beyond the liver, FGF21 analogues improve insulin sensitivity, raise adiponectin, favorably shift the lipid profile, and modestly reduce body weight through central nervous system effects on appetite and energy expenditure.

The Phase 2 clinical trial results have been, by the standards of this disease, striking. In the HARMONY trial of efruxifermin and the ENLIVEN trial of pegozafermin, liver fat reductions on MRI measurement were often dramatic—50 to 70 percent relative reductions, with many participants normalizing liver fat entirely.[349,350] MASH resolution without worsening fibrosis was achieved in 23 to 76 percent of treated patients depending on the trial and dose, compared to substantially lower rates on placebo. Fibrosis improvement of at least one stage was seen in 22 to 49 percent of treated participants versus 7 to 20 percent on placebo—with some signals of benefit even in people with cirrhosis, the most advanced and difficult-to-treat stage. These are biopsy-confirmed histological endpoints, the regulatory gold standard, and the results compare favorably to resmetirom and GLP-1 agonists in meta-analyses for both MASH resolution and fibrosis regression specifically.

FGF21 analogues are not without side effects. Gastrointestinal effects—nausea, diarrhea—and injection-site reactions are the most commonly reported adverse effects in trials to date. The longer-term safety picture, particularly for bone metabolism and cardiovascular outcomes, is still being characterized in ongoing Phase 3 trials. These drugs are not yet approved and are not currently available outside of clinical trial settings. But among the agents in the MASLD pipeline, FGF21 analogues represent one of the most mechanistically compelling and clinically encouraging classes in development—particularly for people with advanced fibrosis, where the combination of potent anti-fibrotic, anti-inflammatory, and metabolic effects addresses the disease at a stage where most other approaches have limited reach.

Pan-PPAR agonists (lanifibranor and others): To understand why pan-PPAR agonists are generating serious clinical interest, it helps to understand what the three PPAR receptors actually do—and why activating only one of them at a time has historically produced incomplete results.

PPAR stands for peroxisome proliferator-activated receptor. Think of the three PPAR isoforms as three separate control panels governing different aspects of the metabolic dysfunction that drives MASLD. PPAR-alpha, expressed predominantly in the liver, is the lipid oxidizer—it upregulates the genes responsible for breaking down fatty acids in the mitochondria and promotes the clearance of fat stored in liver cells. Activating it alone is what fibrate medications do, and fibrates do reduce triglycerides, but their effects on MASH histology have been modest. PPAR-delta, found in the liver, muscle, and adipose tissue, is the metabolic engine—it improves insulin sensitivity, enhances glucose utilization, and suppresses the activation of Kupffer cells, the liver's resident immune cells that are central to the inflammatory cascade of MASH. PPAR-gamma, most prominently expressed in fat tissue, is the insulin sensitizer and fat redistributor—it boosts adiponectin production (a hormone with direct anti-fibrotic effects in the liver), and critically, it redirects fat storage toward subcutaneous depots and away from the liver and viscera, reducing the lipotoxic burden on hepatocytes. This is the receptor activated by pioglitazone, which is why pioglitazone works for MASH but causes weight gain and fluid retention—PPAR-gamma activation alone, at the doses required for meaningful liver benefit, produces those trade-offs reliably.

Pan-PPAR agonists activate all three receptors concurrently, with the goal of achieving the combined benefits of each pathway while using lower relative activation of each receptor than would be required for any single-isoform agent to work alone—potentially reducing the side effects associated with high-dose single-receptor stimulation.[351,352] The result, when it works as designed, is simultaneous fat clearance from the liver via PPAR-alpha, metabolic and anti-inflammatory improvement via

PPAR-delta, and insulin sensitization with fat redistribution via PPAR-gamma. The combined activation also suppresses hepatic stellate cell activity—us suppressing fibrosis—through multiple converging pathways, addressing scarring directly rather than as a downstream consequence of reduced inflammation alone.

The most clinically advanced pan-PPAR agonist is lanifibranor, which completed a Phase 2b trial (NATIVE) in people with biopsy-confirmed MASH.[353] Results were encouraging: the drug produced significant improvements in the composite liver histology score, meaningful reductions in liver fat, and favorable signals for both MASH resolution and fibrosis improvement compared to a placebo. A Phase 3 trial is ongoing. The side effect profile in Phase 2 was notable for peripheral edema—fluid retention in the limbs, consistent with the PPAR-gamma component's effect on sodium and water handling—and modest weight gain, also attributable to PPAR-gamma activation, though both appeared less pronounced than typically seen with pioglitazone alone. Gastrointestinal effects including nausea and diarrhea were reported, as with most agents in the metabolic drug space. Anemia was observed in some participants and warrants monitoring, possibly related to PPAR-delta's effects on hematopoietic signaling.

What is not yet known is more significant than what is. The long-term safety profile of sustained pan-PPAR activation across all three isoforms in humans has not been characterized beyond the relatively short duration of Phase 2 exposure. The cardiovascular implications of prolonged PPAR-delta activation in a population already at elevated cardiovascular risk require careful Phase 3 evaluation—PPAR-delta's role in modulating lipid metabolism, cardiac energy use, and vascular inflammation is complex enough that the long-term cardiovascular signal could be favorable, neutral, or concerning, and current data does not resolve that question. The bone density implications of combined PPAR-gamma and PPAR-alpha activation over years—a concern already documented with thiazolidinediones—have not been adequately studied at pan-PPAR doses. And the question of how pan-PPAR agonism interacts with other medications commonly used in the MASLD population—statins, GLP-1 agonists, antihypertensives—requires longer-term pharmacovigilance data that Phase 2 trials cannot provide. As with FGF21 analogues, the Phase 2 efficacy signal is genuinely encouraging; what Phase 3 trials and eventual post-marketing surveillance will determine is whether the benefit-risk profile holds across a larger, more diverse, and longer-treated population.

Combination approaches: The recognition that MASLD is a multi-mechanism disease is driving interest in combination pharmacotherapy—pairing agents with complementary mechanisms to address more of the disease biology simultaneously, in the same way that combination lifestyle interventions do.

The trajectory of this pipeline suggests that the pharmacological management of MASLD will look considerably different in five to ten years than it does today. The medications most likely to be most effective will be those used alongside—not instead of—the lifestyle behaviors that address the root causes no drug can fully replicate.

How to Have a Productive Conversation with Your Doctor

Many people with fatty liver disease feel passive in clinical conversations about medication—receiving recommendations without fully understanding the rationale, or leaving the appointment with questions they did not think to ask. A more active, informed approach produces better outcomes and a better therapeutic relationship.

The following questions are worth raising in any conversation where medication for fatty liver disease is being considered:

- **"What is my current disease stage, and does the evidence support medication at this stage?"** Not everyone with fatty liver disease is at a stage where pharmaceutical intervention is guideline-supported. Understanding where you are on the spectrum—simple steatosis, early MASH, MASH with fibrosis—clarifies whether a medication conversation is timely or premature.
- **"What specific outcome is this medication expected to produce, and over what timeframe?"** Goals matter. Is the aim to reduce liver fat, improve fibrosis, lower liver enzymes, improve glycemic control, or reduce cardiovascular risk? Knowing the target and the expected timeline for achieving it allows you to evaluate whether the medication is working.
- **"What are the most common and most serious side effects, and how will we monitor for them?"** A complete side effect discussion—not just the most common mild effects but the serious ones relevant to your specific health situation—is part of informed consent. Do not leave this to the package insert.
- **"How does this medication interact with my lifestyle changes, and will I need to continue medication indefinitely?"** Understanding the relationship between the drug and the lifestyle work you are doing—and what happens if the medication is eventually stopped—is essential for setting realistic expectations and planning appropriately.

- **"Are there less expensive or better-established alternatives given my specific situation?"** Newer is not always better, and the cost of newer branded medications is a real barrier for many people. Pioglitazone, vitamin E (in appropriate candidates), and off-label use of SGLT2 inhibitors or GLP-1 agonists may offer meaningful benefit at lower cost or with a more established safety record for some individuals.

Start Here: Your Medication Decision Framework

Step 1 — Establish Your Current Stage

- Confirm with your doctor whether you have simple steatosis, MASH without fibrosis, or MASH with fibrosis—and at what stage. Medication decisions are stage-dependent.
- If you have not had a FibroScan or liver biopsy and your disease stage is uncertain, ask whether noninvasive fibrosis assessment is appropriate for your situation.

Step 2 — Give Lifestyle Its Full Chance First

- This step is not a formality. The scientific evidence is clear: Consistent dietary change, regular resistance and aerobic exercise, targeted sleep improvement, stress management, and the strategic supplementation discussed in Chapters 9 and 10 produce meaningful, measurable liver improvements in most people with early-stage MASLD. Six to twelve months of genuine, consistent implementation—not halfhearted attempts alongside unchanged eating habits—is the appropriate trial period before concluding that lifestyle is insufficient.
- Many people discover in this process that their liver enzymes normalize, their fibrosis markers stabilize, and their metabolic markers shift significantly—without any

pharmaceutical involvement. That is not an anecdote; it is the expected outcome of well-implemented lifestyle change at early disease stages.

- If you are early in your lifestyle change journey, this step is your whole current assignment. Come back to the rest of this framework when you have genuinely given the foundation time to work.

Step 3 — Consider Your Full Metabolic Picture

- Do you have type 2 diabetes or prediabetes? GLP-1 agonists or SGLT2 inhibitors may address both conditions simultaneously.
- Do you have significant cardiovascular risk or established cardiovascular disease? SGLT2 inhibitors have the strongest cardiovascular mortality data and a liver benefit signal.
- Do you have biopsy-confirmed MASH with fibrosis stage 2 or above? Resmetirom is now FDA-approved for this specific indication.
- Are you nondiabetic with biopsy-confirmed MASH? Pioglitazone and vitamin E both have relevant evidence in this population.

Step 4 — Monitor and Reassess

- Any medication added to your protocol should have a defined reassessment point—typically three to six months—at which liver enzymes, metabolic markers, and if appropriate, imaging are reviewed to confirm the medication is producing the expected benefit.
- If a medication is not producing meaningful benefit at adequate doses after an appropriate trial period, continuing it is not automatically justified. Side effects, cost, and lack of efficacy in a specific individual are all legitimate reasons to reassess.

- Medication is not a one-way door. Starting it does not commit you to continuing it indefinitely, particularly if your liver health improves to a point where the risk-benefit calculation changes.

> ***The Overarching Principle.*** *Every medication discussed in this chapter works best when lifestyle is working alongside it. The drugs that produce the most dramatic results in clinical trials are the ones studied in populations that also received dietary counseling, exercise guidance, and structured support for behavior change. The lifestyle foundation is not the consolation prize for people who cannot access medication. It is the platform on which medication, when appropriate, performs at its best.*

Key Takeaways

- **For the majority of people with early-stage MASLD, lifestyle change is sufficient.** Consistent dietary improvement, regular exercise, targeted supplementation, sleep optimization, and stress management address the root causes of fatty liver disease in ways no medication can fully replicate—and produce lasting results that do not reverse when the intervention stops. Medications are most relevant in confirmed MASH with fibrosis, in people whose disease has not adequately responded to sustained lifestyle intervention, and in those with significant metabolic comorbidities requiring pharmaceutical management for independent reasons.

- Medications are most relevant in confirmed MASH with fibrosis, in people whose disease has not adequately responded to sustained lifestyle intervention, and in those with significant metabolic comorbidities where pharmaceutical management of those conditions simultaneously benefits the liver.

- GLP-1 receptor agonists (semaglutide, liraglutide) produce documented and meaningful reductions in liver fat, MASH resolution, and fibrosis improvement—but carry a significant and underreported side effect profile including gastroparesis, pancreatitis, gallbladder disease, potential mood effects, thyroid concerns, and near-universal weight regain upon discontinuation without sustained lifestyle change.

- Pioglitazone has one of the longest evidence records for MASH and is particularly relevant for people with concurrent type 2 diabetes, with consistent histological improvement in trials—but causes weight gain, fluid retention, and carries bone fracture and potential bladder cancer considerations.

- Resmetirom is the first FDA-approved drug specifically for MASH with fibrosis, demonstrating genuine histological benefit through selective thyroid hormone receptor beta activation. It is a meaningful advance and an appropriate conversation to have with a hepatologist for people with moderate to advanced fibrosis.

- SGLT2 inhibitors benefit the liver through insulin-independent glucose clearance, visceral fat reduction, and direct hepatic effects—most clearly established in people with concurrent type 2 diabetes or cardiovascular disease.

- Statins are underused in MASLD due to a largely unfounded fear of liver toxicity. They should be discussed with an integrative-minded physician who clearly understands the risks-benefit calculation and only when truly medically warranted.

With the clinical and pharmaceutical landscape fully mapped, the final chapter brings the entire strategy together. Chapter 12 looks at where the science of fatty liver disease is heading, what emerging technologies and precision approaches will mean for future management, and how to build the kind of lifelong liver health plan that sustains the gains you have made—and continues to protect you for decades to come.

CHAPTER 12

The Future of Fatty Liver Disease

Innovation, Prevention, and Building a Liver-Healthy Life

There is a version of this chapter that reads like a technology brochure. AI-powered diagnostics. Microbiome sequencing. Personalized nutrition algorithms. Smart wearables that track your metabolic state in real time. Precision medicine that tailors treatment to your specific genetic profile. All of it is real, all of it is developing, and some of it will meaningfully change how fatty liver disease is detected, managed, and eventually prevented at a population level.

But technology does not eat breakfast. Algorithms do not take a walk at lunch. Precision medicine cannot make up for a life built around ultra-processed food, chronic sleep deprivation, and unmanaged stress. The most sophisticated diagnostic tool in the world is of limited value if what it finds is not then acted upon.

This final chapter looks forward honestly—at the genuinely exciting developments in detection, personalization, and emerging therapy—while returning, one last time, to the foundational truth that has run through every page of this book: The most powerful intervention available for fatty liver disease is the one you execute consistently, starting today. The future of medicine will offer remarkable new tools. The foundation on which those tools work best is the one you are building right now.

Precision Medicine: From Population Averages to Individual Profiles

Most of the research discussed in this book presents population-level findings: On average, people who do X see Y improvement. That framing is scientifically necessary and clinically useful, but it glosses over something every person with fatty liver disease eventually notices—the same intervention produces dramatically different results in different people.

Two people follow the same Mediterranean diet for twelve weeks. One achieves a 40 percent reduction in liver fat. The other achieves 12 percent. Same diet, same duration, meaningfully different outcomes. The explanation lies in the differences between them—their genetic variants affecting fat metabolism, their baseline microbiome composition, their specific pattern of insulin resistance, their hormonal environment, their sleep architecture, their individual response to dietary carbohydrate. These are not noise in the data. They are the signal that precision medicine is designed to interpret.

The field of precision nutrition—tailoring dietary recommendations to the individual's genetic, metabolic, and microbiome profile rather than applying universal guidelines—is advancing rapidly. Pioneering research from the Weizmann Institute, led by Eran Segal and his colleagues, demonstrated that different individuals show dramatically different blood sugar responses to identical foods, driven largely by microbiome composition and individual metabolic factors.[354] Personalized dietary recommendations based on these profiles produced significantly better glycemic outcomes than standard nutritional guidelines—a finding with direct implications for fatty liver disease management, where blood sugar and insulin control are central.

Genetic testing for MASLD risk variants—particularly PNPLA3, TM6SF2, and MBOAT7—is moving toward clinical utility.[355] Knowing your genetic risk profile does not change the foundational lifestyle approach, but it does sharpen the urgency of implementing it and may eventually inform more targeted pharmaceutical decisions. People carrying high-risk PNPLA3 variants, for example, appear to derive particular benefit from omega-3 fatty acid supplementation—a gene-nutrient interaction that population-level guidelines cannot capture but personalized medicine will. However, the research is ongoing and not fully conclusive.

The practical implication for most people today is modest but meaningful: Microbiome testing, continuous glucose monitoring (CGM), and genetic testing are all becoming more accessible and less expensive. None of them is required to follow the approach in this book—the foundational lifestyle strategies benefit virtually everyone regardless of their individual profile. But for people whose response to standard interventions has been unexpectedly limited, these tools can identify the specific biological factors that explain why and point toward more targeted solutions.

Digital Health Tools: Technology in Service of Behavior

The gap between knowing what to do and consistently doing it is where most health interventions fail. Digital health tools—when well-designed and thoughtfully used—are among the most promising developments for closing that gap.

Continuous Glucose Monitors

Continuous glucose monitors, originally developed for people with diabetes, are increasingly used by metabolically healthy individuals and those with prediabetes or MASLD to gain real-time insight into how their bodies respond to specific foods, meal timing, exercise, sleep, and stress. A CGM worn for two to four weeks can answer questions that no standard blood test can: How does my blood sugar respond to a smoothie versus eggs for breakfast? How much does a thirty-minute walk after dinner blunt my post-meal glucose spike? How does a poor night's sleep affect my fasting glucose the following morning?

This kind of personalized, real-time metabolic feedback is genuinely transformative for many people. It converts abstract nutritional advice into concrete, personalized data—making the connection between specific behaviors and metabolic consequences visible in a way that changes decision-making. Research on CGM use in nondiabetic metabolic disease populations consistently shows improvements in dietary quality, insulin sensitivity, and engagement with lifestyle change.[356] For people with MASLD who are motivated to understand their individual metabolic responses rather than simply following generic guidelines, a short-term CGM trial is one of the highest-value health technology investments currently available.

Digital Therapeutics and Behavioral Support

Smartphone-based interventions for lifestyle change in metabolic disease have moved well beyond simple calorie-counting apps. Digital therapeutics—software programs that deliver evidence-based behavioral health interventions—have demonstrated meaningful clinical outcomes in randomized controlled trials for type 2 diabetes, hypertension, and obesity.[357] Programs that combine dietary tracking, personalized coaching, educational content, and community support produce improvements in HbA1c, body weight, and metabolic markers comparable to structured in-person programs—at a fraction of the cost and with far greater scalability.

For fatty liver disease specifically, several digital programs targeting the metabolic components of MASLD are in development or early deployment, some integrated with CGM data and some with direct hepatology oversight. The evidence base for these programs is early but directionally consistent: Structured digital support for behavior change outperforms no support, and the accountability and feedback mechanisms embedded in well-designed apps reduce the adherence gap that derails so many lifestyle interventions.

The caveat is quality. The app stores contain thousands of health and nutrition applications, the overwhelming majority of which are not grounded in evidence and some of which promote approaches actively harmful to metabolic health. Seek programs that cite their clinical evidence base, that are designed with input from qualified clinicians, and that provide personalized feedback rather than one-size-fits-all prescriptions.

Wearables and Metabolic Tracking

Wearable devices—smartwatches, fitness trackers, sleep monitors—now capture data that was previously accessible only in clinical research settings: continuous heart rate variability (a proxy for autonomic nervous system balance, vagal tone, and stress recovery), sleep stage architecture, activity levels and non-exercise activity thermogenesis (NEAT), resting heart rate trends, and blood oxygen saturation. The clinical utility of this data for MASLD management is still being established, but several signals are already practically useful.

Heart rate variability (HRV) tracking, in particular, provides a real-time window into the balance between sympathetic and parasympathetic nervous system activity—the same cortisol-recovery dynamic discussed in Chapter 7. Consistently low HRV is a reliable early indicator of accumulated physiological stress, inadequate sleep recovery, or overtraining, all of which translate directly to worsened insulin sensitivity and metabolic health. Using HRV data to guide the balance between training intensity and recovery—backing off when HRV trends downward, progressing when it is elevated—is one of the most practically evidence-informed uses of wearable data currently available.

Sleep tracking data, while imperfect in its accuracy for specific sleep stages, provides trends that are meaningfully useful over time. Consistent documentation of sleep duration, sleep timing consistency, and disrupted nights provides both accountability and early warning when the sleep patterns established in Chapter 7 are slipping.

AI and Early Detection: Finding the Disease Before It Progresses

One of the most significant challenges in fatty liver disease management has always been that most people do not know they have it until it has already progressed. Routine liver function tests miss a substantial proportion of cases. Ultrasound requires a trained operator and has variable sensitivity. Liver biopsy—the diagnostic gold standard—is invasive, expensive, and carries procedural risk. The result is a disease that is massively underdiagnosed at the stage where intervention is most effective.

Artificial intelligence is beginning to change this. Machine learning algorithms trained on large datasets of clinical, laboratory, imaging, and demographic data can now identify individuals at high risk for MASLD and MASH with accuracy that rivals specialist clinical assessment—using data that is already routinely collected. A patient's age, BMI, fasting glucose, triglycerides, ALT, platelet count, and a handful of other standard laboratory values, fed into an appropriately trained algorithm, can generate a probabilistic MASLD risk score that flags individuals who should receive further evaluation. Several such algorithms are being integrated into electronic health record systems, generating automated alerts when a patient's routine bloodwork pattern suggests undiagnosed fatty liver disease.

AI-assisted analysis of liver ultrasound and CT imaging is also advancing rapidly. Algorithms trained on thousands of annotated liver images can detect subtle changes in liver echogenicity, texture, and morphology that human readers might miss—improving both sensitivity and consistency of fatty liver detection from standard imaging modalities that are already widely used. More sophisticated applications are beginning to estimate liver fat percentage and fibrosis stage from routine CT scans without the need for dedicated MRI or biopsy.

Noninvasive fibrosis assessment is another area of rapid progress. FIB-4 score—a simple formula using age, ALT, AST, and platelet count—is already validated and widely recommended as a first-line triage tool.[358] Enhanced liver fibrosis (ELF) panels, combining serum markers of fibrosis activity, improve on this further. FibroScan (transient elastography), which measures liver stiffness as a proxy for fibrosis, is becoming more widely available in primary care and specialist settings. The direction of travel is clear: The need for liver biopsy to stage disease will diminish as noninvasive tools become more accurate and more accessible, lowering the threshold for early identification and earlier intervention.

For people reading this book, the practical implication is to advocate for appropriate screening. If you have metabolic syndrome, type 2 diabetes, significant obesity, or even a cluster of risk factors—elevated triglycerides, low HDL, elevated fasting glucose, and central obesity—requesting a FIB-4 calculation, a FibroScan, or at minimum a liver ultrasound is a reasonable and increasingly guideline-supported conversation to have with your doctor. The window for intervention is widest when the disease is found early. Better tools for finding it early are arriving, and using them is part of a proactive approach to your own health.

The Public Health Picture: Why Individual Action Exists in a Broader Context

Fatty liver disease at a population level is not primarily a failure of individual willpower. It is the predictable metabolic consequence of a food environment engineered for palatability and profit, a built environment that makes sedentary behavior the path of least resistance, work cultures that treat sleep deprivation as productivity, and chronic economic and social stressors that activate the cortisol pathways described in Chapter 7 for millions of people simultaneously.

This is not a counsel of helplessness—it is an accurate description of why individual effort, while necessary and genuinely powerful, operates within a context that either supports or undermines it. Understanding this context matters for two reasons. First, it should reduce the self-blame that many people with metabolic disease carry unnecessarily. Developing fatty liver disease in the modern world is not primarily a character failure. Second, it points toward the kinds of systemic changes—food labeling reform, reduction of ultra-processed food marketing to children, urban design that prioritizes walkability, workplace policies that protect sleep and reduce chronic stress—that will ultimately determine whether MASLD rates decline at a population level rather than merely in the individuals who read books like this one.

You cannot wait for those systemic changes before acting on your own health. But you can hold both truths at once: that your individual choices matter enormously, and that they are made harder than they should be by an environment that was not designed with your metabolic health in mind. Give yourself appropriate credit for the effort required to swim upstream—and extend the same generosity to others you know who are struggling.

The MASLD Reversal Blueprint: Your Whole Strategy at a Glance

Eleven chapters of science, mechanisms, strategies, and practical tools now sit behind you. Before moving to the closing reflection, it is worth crystallizing the entire approach into its essential architecture—the integrated framework that makes every individual strategy more effective than it would be in isolation.

The Foundation – Non-Negotiable

- **Nutrition:** Reduce sugar-sweetened beverages and ultra-processed foods. Eat in a Mediterranean-style pattern centered on vegetables, legumes, fatty fish, olive oil, and whole foods. Consider time-restricted eating aligned with daylight hours. Adequate protein at every meal.
- **Movement:** Daily aerobic activity building toward 150 minutes per week. Resistance training two to three times per

week. Hourly movement breaks during sedentary work. More NEAT throughout every day.

- **Sleep:** Seven to nine hours consistently. Fixed wake time. Morning light, evening darkness. Late eating eliminated. Sleep apnea evaluated if suspected.
- **Stress management:** A practiced, daily recovery habit—breathing, mindfulness, nature exposure, or restorative social connection. Not the elimination of stress, but consistent recovery from it.

The Gut-Liver Layer – High Impact, Often Overlooked

- **Microbiome diversity:** Thirty or more different plant foods per week. Prebiotic-rich foods daily. Daily fermented foods. Reduce dietary sugar to starve ethanol-producing gut bacteria.
- **Fiber:** 25 to 35 grams daily from whole food sources, increasing gradually. Resistant starch sources incorporated regularly.
- **Probiotic support:** A high-quality multi-strain probiotic as a daily foundational supplement.

The Supplement Layer – Targeted Support

- **Core:** Optimized vitamin D (40 to 80 ng/mL by testing), omega-3 fatty acids (2 to 4 grams EPA/DHA daily), berberine or myo-inositol for insulin resistance, niacinamide for the microRNA-93/SIRT1 pathway.
- **Liver-supportive:** Silymarin phospholipid complex, enhanced-bioavailability curcumin, artichoke extract where bile and cholesterol are concerns.

- **Hormonal:** Address sex hormone contributors and thyroid function where relevant—these are frequently underdiagnosed limiters on metabolic progress.

The Monitoring Layer – Know Whether It's Working

- **Baseline labs:** ALT, AST, GGT, fasting glucose, fasting insulin, HOMA-IR, HbA1c, triglycerides, HDL, full lipid panel.
- **Recheck at three and six months:** Confirm that the strategy is producing the expected biological improvements. Adjust based on what the data shows, not just how you feel.
- **Waist circumference monthly:** A more sensitive early indicator of visceral fat change than scale weight.
- **Consider FibroScan or imaging:** At baseline and annually if disease stage is established, to track structural liver changes over time.

The Medical Layer – Where Appropriate

- **Discuss medication:** For confirmed MASH with fibrosis stage 2 or above, for inadequate response to sustained lifestyle effort, or for significant comorbidities where pharmaceutical management offers simultaneous metabolic and liver benefit.
- **Stay current:** The pharmaceutical landscape for MASLD is changing faster than almost any other therapeutic area. The conversation with your hepatologist or gastroenterologist in two years will include options that do not exist today.

Building a Lifelong Liver Health Plan

The word "reversal" in the context of fatty liver disease is accurate and appropriate for most people reading this book—but it can inadvertently imply a finish line that does not exist. The lifestyle that reverses fatty liver disease is not a temporary program with a defined endpoint. It is a permanent redefinition of how you live.

This does not mean permanent austerity or joyless restriction. The Mediterranean pattern of eating is one of the most pleasurable, culturally rich, and varied ways of eating on the planet. Strength training, when it becomes a genuine habit, is one of the most reliably mood-enhancing behaviors available. Seven to eight hours of sleep is not a sacrifice—it is a restoration. Managed stress and the parasympathetic recovery it enables does not diminish life. It expands the capacity to live it.

What changes permanently is the orientation. The question is no longer "Can I get away with this?" but "Does this serve the metabolic health I am building?" That is not a burden. It is a framework. And frameworks, unlike diets, do not end.

The research on long-term liver health outcomes is clear: people who maintain the lifestyle changes that produced initial liver improvement sustain those improvements. People who return to the patterns that drove the disease in the first place see their liver fat and metabolic markers return. The liver is responsive in both directions, and it is continuously reflecting the cumulative average of the inputs it receives. This is not a threat—it is the most empowering finding in the entire field. Your liver is listening. It responds to what you do. And it will continue to respond for as long as you continue to give it what it needs. You are generally a reflection of your diet, lifestyle, and environment.

What to Do Today

Every chapter in this book has ended with a practical starting point. This one is no different—except that the starting point is the entire strategy, distilled to its most essential first actions.

- **If you have not yet had baseline labs, request them at your next appointment.** ALT, AST, fasting insulin, triglycerides, HbA1c, and vitamin D. You cannot navigate without a map.
- **If you are still drinking sugar-sweetened beverages regularly, stop today.** Not gradually. Today. This single change begins reducing liver fat faster than almost any other dietary intervention, requires no new skills, costs nothing (in fact it saves money), and produces measurable biological improvement within weeks.
- **If you are not moving daily, take a twenty-minute walk today.** Not a structured program. Not a gym membership. A walk. The dose-response curve for exercise and liver health is steepest in the transition from sedentary to lightly active, and a walk is where that transition begins.
- **If you are consistently sleeping fewer than seven hours, commit tonight to a fixed wake time and protect it.** The hormonal cascade of chronic sleep deprivation actively undermines everything else you do for your health. No dietary or supplement strategy can fully compensate for it.
- **If you have not told your doctor that improving your liver health is a priority, tell them at your next visit.** Your care team can only support goals they know about. An informed, engaged physician who understands your priorities is a meaningful asset in your long-term management.

None of these actions requires a perfect plan. They require a decision—and then a second one tomorrow, and a third one the day after. The strategy in this book is not built from heroic single efforts. It is built from the accumulation of ordinary, consistent choices made by someone who has decided that their health is worth protecting.

✦ ✦ ✦

Key Takeaways

- Precision medicine—including genetic testing for MASLD risk variants, microbiome profiling, and personalized nutrition algorithms—is advancing toward clinical utility and will increasingly allow lifestyle and pharmaceutical interventions to be tailored to the individual's specific biological profile.
- Digital health tools—CGMs, digital therapeutics, HRV tracking, sleep monitors—are closing the gap between knowing what to do and consistently doing it. Continuous glucose monitoring in particular provides the kind of personalized, real-time metabolic feedback that generic guidelines cannot offer.
- AI-driven early detection—through pattern recognition in routine laboratory and imaging data—is moving fatty liver disease diagnosis upstream toward earlier, more actionable stages of disease. Noninvasive fibrosis assessment is improving rapidly and will increasingly replace biopsy for staging.
- The MASLD pharmaceutical pipeline is the most active in history. FGF21 analogues, pan-PPAR agonists, dual and triple hormone receptor agonists, and combination approaches will substantially expand treatment options over the next five to ten years. The lifestyle foundation that makes

these tools most effective will remain constant regardless of which drugs become available.

- Fatty liver disease at a population level reflects a food and lifestyle environment that is poorly aligned with human metabolic health. Individual effort is both necessary and genuinely powerful—and it is made harder than it should be by systemic factors that are not a personal failing.
- The lifestyle that reverses fatty liver disease is not a temporary program. It is a permanent reorientation—one that, when built thoughtfully and sustained consistently, becomes less about discipline and more about identity.
- The liver responds to the cumulative average of the inputs it receives—continuously, in both directions. This is not a warning. It is the most empowering fact in metabolic medicine.

A Final Word

When you received the news about your liver—whether from a routine blood test, an incidental ultrasound finding, or a more deliberate diagnostic workup—you likely felt some version of what most people feel: confusion, concern, perhaps a quiet dread about what it might mean.

What you may not have felt, in that moment, is what this book has tried to give you: clarity. The knowledge that what you are dealing with has a name, a mechanism, and a set of well-characterized, evidence-grounded responses that genuinely work. That the organ in question is one of the most regenerative in the human body. That the disease, for most people, is caught at a stage where meaningful reversal is not only possible but probable with consistent effort. That the same lifestyle choices that protect the liver also protect the heart, the brain, the kidneys, the hormonal system, and the quality of every year of life ahead.

The strategies in this book are not experimental. They are not extreme. They are the accumulated findings of decades of rigorous science, translated into the most practical, accessible, and sustainable form possible. They do not require perfection. They require consistency. They do not require suffering. They require intention—and then the daily practice of acting on it.

You now have the understanding of what MASLD is and why it develops. You have the nutritional framework to eat in a way that actively repairs rather than burdens your liver. You have the exercise science to move in a way that heals hepatic tissue independently of the scale. You have the sleep and stress tools to restore the hormonal environment in which metabolic healing can occur. You have the gut health strategies to address the microbiome-liver connection that so many approaches overlook. You have a clear, evidence-grounded supplement protocol. You have an honest account of the pharmaceutical options and when they are appropriate. And you have a picture of where the science is heading—so that as new tools become available, you will understand how to use them wisely.

What you do with all of that is, of course, up to you. But the path is clear, the science is sound, and the outcome—for those who walk it consistently—is well-established.

Following the guidance in this book will help you beat fatty liver disease naturally.

APPENDIX A

Sample 7-Day Liver-Friendly Meal Plan

This meal plan applies the nutritional principles from Chapter 4: Mediterranean-style eating, reduced refined carbohydrates and added sugars, adequate protein at every meal, abundant fiber, two to three servings of fatty fish per week, and eating windows that close by 7 PM where possible. It is a flexible framework, not a rigid prescription. Substitute freely within the same food categories based on preference, availability, and cultural tradition.

> *Key principles at a glance: no sugar-sweetened beverages at any meal; olive oil as the primary cooking fat; fermented foods included daily (yogurt, kefir, sauerkraut); coffee or green tea without added sugar; water as the default beverage.*

Meal	What to Eat
Day 1 — Monday	
Breakfast	Two scrambled eggs in olive oil with spinach and tomatoes · Half avocado · Water, black coffee, or green tea
Snack	Small handful of walnuts · 1 cup plain Greek yogurt with a few blueberries

Lunch	Large salad: mixed greens, chickpeas, cucumber, cherry tomatoes, red onion · Olive oil and lemon dressing · Canned sardines or grilled salmon alongside
Snack	Vegetable sticks (celery, bell pepper) with hummus
Dinner	Baked salmon with garlic and lemon · Roasted broccoli with olive oil · Small serving of lentils or quinoa · Finish by 7 PM
Day 2 — Tuesday	
Breakfast	Organic steel-cut oats with mixed berries, a tablespoon of ground flaxseed, and a sprinkle of cinnamon · Hard-boiled egg alongside · Water or green tea
Snack	Apple slices with almond butter
Lunch	Lentil soup with crusty whole-grain bread · Side salad with olive oil and vinegar
Snack	Plain kefir (small glass) · Handful of almonds
Dinner	Chicken thighs roasted with garlic, turmeric, and olive oil · Steamed green beans · Roasted sweet potato (small)
Day 3 — Wednesday	
Breakfast	Smoked salmon on one slice whole-grain sourdough toast · Sliced cucumber and capers · Water or black coffee
Snack	Small bowl of mixed berries · 10–12 walnuts
Lunch	Whole-grain wrap with grilled chicken, avocado, spinach, and tomato · Sparkling water with lemon
Snack	Carrot sticks and tahini
Dinner	Mackerel or trout pan-seared in olive oil · Sautéed kale with garlic · Cooked chickpeas tossed with lemon and olive oil

Day 4 — Thursday	
Breakfast	Two-egg omelet with diced peppers, onion, and feta · Side of fresh fruit (berries or orange) · Water or green tea
Snack	Greek yogurt with a drizzle of olive oil and a few walnuts
Lunch	Quinoa bowl: quinoa, roasted vegetables (zucchini, bell pepper, eggplant), tahini dressing, fresh herbs
Snack	Small handful of mixed nuts and seeds
Dinner	Tempeh stir-fried with broccoli, snap peas, garlic, and ginger in sesame and olive oil · Brown rice (small serving)

Day 5 — Friday	
Breakfast	Full-fat plain yogurt parfait: yogurt, mixed berries, ground flaxseed, and a few pumpkin seeds · Water or black coffee
Snack	Two hard-boiled eggs · Sliced cucumber
Lunch	Tuna salad (olive oil, lemon, capers, red onion) on a bed of mixed greens and avocado
Snack	Sauerkraut alongside a small serving of cottage cheese
Dinner	Baked white fish (cod or sea bass) with herb crust · Roasted asparagus and cherry tomatoes · Side of white beans with garlic and lemon

Day 6 — Saturday	
Breakfast	Vegetable frittata with eggs, spinach, mushrooms, and onion cooked in olive oil · Fresh fruit · Water or green tea
Snack	Kefir smoothie: kefir, frozen berries, spinach, ground flaxseed, half a banana
Lunch	Mediterranean mezze plate: hummus, tabbouleh, olives, feta, sliced cucumber, whole-grain pita (small)

Snack	Dark chocolate (85%+, small square) · Handful of almonds
Dinner	Grilled lamb or beef kebabs (modest serving) with tzatziki · Roasted root vegetables · Large Greek salad
Day 7 — Sunday	
Breakfast	Avocado toast on whole-grain sourdough · Poached eggs · Sliced tomato with olive oil and sea salt · Water or black coffee
Snack	Apple and a small wedge of Swiss cheese
Lunch	Minestrone soup with white beans, tomatoes, kale, and whole-grain pasta (small amount) · Side of crusty bread
Snack	Plain Greek yogurt with a few berries and a drizzle of honey (small amount)
Dinner	Roasted salmon with fennel and orange slices · Wilted spinach with garlic and olive oil · Green lentils · Finish by 7 PM

Notes on flexibility: Proteins are interchangeable within type (any fatty fish for salmon; any legume for chickpeas; eggs for meat at breakfast). Vegetables are fully interchangeable. The pattern—not the exact foods—is what matters. Aim for 25 to 30 different plant foods across the week.

APPENDIX B

Exercise Templates

Beginner Template – Weeks 1 Through 8

Start here if you are currently sedentary or have not exercised regularly in the past year. No gym membership or equipment is required for the first four weeks. The priority is establishing a consistent daily movement habit before increasing intensity or volume.

Exercise	Sets × Reps	Notes
WEEK 1–2: ESTABLISH THE HABIT (3 days/week — Mon / Wed / Fri)		
Brisk walk	1 × 20 min	Pace where breathing is elevated but you can still speak in sentences. Outdoors preferred.
Air squats	2 × 10	Feet shoulder-width apart, chest up, lower until thighs approach parallel. Pause at bottom.
Wall push-ups	2 × 8–10	Hands on wall at chest height. Build to floor push-ups over weeks 3–4.
Seated or standing calf raises	2 × 12	Use a step edge for fuller range of motion if available.

Dead bug (core)	2 × 8 each side	Lie on back, arms up, extend opposite arm/leg while keeping lower back flat on floor.
Hourly movement break	2–3 min every hour	Stand up, walk to another room, do 10 air squats, or march in place. Non-negotiable on sedentary workdays.
WEEK 3–4: BUILD DURATION AND ADD RESISTANCE		
Brisk walk	1 × 25–30 min	Extend duration. Add a short uphill section if available.
Bodyweight squats	3 × 12	Add a 2-second pause at the bottom to increase time under tension.
Push-ups (floor)	2 × 8–10	Transition from wall if ready. Knees-down variation is fine—form over depth.
Resistance band rows	3 × 10	Anchor band at chest height; pull elbows back, squeeze shoulder blades together.
Glute bridges	3 × 12	Lie on back, feet flat, drive hips up. Hold 2 seconds at top.
Plank hold	3 × 15–20 sec	Elbows under shoulders, body in a straight line. Increase hold time by 5 seconds each week.

WEEK 5–8: PROGRESS AND CONSOLIDATE (4 days/week)		
Aerobic activity	4 × 30 min/week	Vary modalities: walking, cycling, swimming, or any preferred aerobic activity.
Goblet squat (with weight)	3 × 12	Hold a dumbbell or kettlebell at chest. Increase loading safely for beginners.
Push-up progression	3 × 10–12	Work toward full push-ups. Add a slow (3-second) lowering phase for added benefit.
Dumbbell row	3 × 10 each side	Brace on bench or chair. Pull dumbbell to hip, not shoulder. Control the lowering.
Reverse lunges	3 × 10 each leg	Step back rather than forward—easier on the knee joint for beginners.
Dead bug or bird dog	3 × 10 each side	Alternate sides. Slow and controlled. Core bracing throughout.

Intermediate Template – For Established Exercisers

Use this template if you already exercise occasionally but want a structured program optimized for liver and metabolic health. Requires access to dumbbells or a gym. Perform Day A and Day B twice each per week on nonconsecutive days (e.g., Mon/Thu and Tue/Fri).

Exercise	Sets × Reps	Notes
DAY A — LOWER BODY + CORE (repeat 2×/week with 48 hrs rest between)		
Goblet squat or barbell back squat	4 × 8–10	Progressive overload: Increase weight by the smallest available increment when you can complete all reps with good form.
Romanian deadlift	3 × 10	Hip hinge, not a squat. Soft knee, neutral spine. Feel the hamstring stretch at the bottom.
Walking lunges	3 × 12 each leg	Add dumbbells when bodyweight feels easy. Keep torso upright.
Hip thrust (barbell or dumbbell)	3 × 12	Upper back on bench, drive through heels. One of the best glute and posterior chain exercises available.
Plank—three variations	3 × 30–45 sec	Standard, side plank (each side), and RKC plank (squeeze everything). Rotate each session.

Dead bug	3 × 10 each side	Slow, controlled. Exhale on extension. Do not let lower back arch off floor.
DAY B — UPPER BODY + METABOLIC (repeat 2×/week alternating with Day A)		
Dumbbell bench press or push-up variation	4 × 8–10	Slow lowering (3 seconds) increases time under tension without requiring heavier weight.
Dumbbell or cable row	4 × 10	Full retraction of shoulder blade at top. Avoid shrugging.
Overhead press (dumbbell or barbell)	3 × 8–10	Brace core throughout. Press in a slight forward arc, not straight up.
Lat pulldown or assisted pull-up	3 × 10	Pull to upper chest, not behind the neck. Elbows down and back.
Dumbbell bicep curl	2 × 12	Supinate (twist palm up) through the full range of motion.
Triceps dips or pushdown	2 × 12	Control the lowering phase. Avoid excessive shoulder internal rotation.
WEEKLY AEROBIC COMPONENT (all levels)		
Moderate aerobic activity	3–4 × 30–40 min	Walking, cycling, swimming, rowing. Conversational pace—you can speak in sentences but breathing is elevated.
Optional HIIT session	1 × 15–20 min	20–30 sec high effort / 60–90 sec easy recovery × 8–10 rounds. Replace one aerobic

		session per week. Not for beginners.
Daily step target	7,000–10,000 steps	Measured by phone or wearable. Treat as a minimum floor, not a ceiling.
Hourly movement breaks	2–3 min / hour	10–15 air squats or a brief walk. Continue regardless of formal exercise completed that day.

Progressive overload principle: Each week, attempt to add either one repetition per set or a small amount of weight to at least one exercise. Over months, this accumulated progression is what builds muscle mass and metabolic capacity. Record your weights—you cannot manage what you do not measure.

APPENDIX C

Supplement Quick-Reference Guide

This guide summarizes the supplements discussed in Chapter 9 in a practical reference format. All doses are general evidence-based ranges for adults; individual needs vary. Always discuss supplement additions with your healthcare provider, particularly if you are taking medications. Begin with Tier 1 supplements and add others based on your specific health profile.

Quality standard: Seek third-party tested products (NSF, USP, Informed Sport, or ConsumerLab certification) and clinically studied branded forms where available. A supplement that does not contain what the label claims, at the dose stated, is not a supplement—it is an expense.

Supplement	Dose & Form	Key Notes & Who Benefits Most
TIER 1 — Strongest Evidence for MASLD		
Omega-3 (EPA/DHA)	2–4 g/day combined EPA+DHA · Fish oil or algae-based	Reduces liver fat, triglycerides, and liver inflammation. Most beneficial when dietary fish intake is low. Choose third-party tested oil with low TOTOX score.

Vitamin E (mixed tocopherols)	400–800 IU/day · d-alpha + gamma tocopherol form	For nondiabetic adults with biopsy-confirmed MASH. Use mixed tocopherol formulation to avoid gamma-tocopherol depletion and associated prostate cancer risk. Discuss with physician first.
Vitamin B3 (Niacinamide)	250–500 mg/day · Niacinamide (nonflushing form preferred)	Suppresses microRNA-93, restoring SIRT1 fat-oxidation pathway. Also raises HDL and lowers triglycerides. Niacinamide avoids flushing at therapeutic doses.
Berberine	900–1,500 mg/day · Divided doses with meals	AMPK activator. Comparable to metformin for insulin resistance and glycemic control. Also improves gut microbiome. Monitor blood sugar if on diabetes medications.
Vitamin D3	Insufficiency or deficiency: 5,000–10,000 IU/day (short-term, monitor labs); Maintenance: 2,000–5,000 IU/day · D3 (cholecalciferol) with a fat-containing meal	Test first. Target serum level 40–60 ng/mL. Deficiency strongly associated with worse MASLD outcomes. Nearly universal benefit—most people are insufficient.

Myo-Inositol	2–4 g/day myo-inositol · Ideally 40:1 myo- to D-chiro-inositol ratio	Second-messenger insulin signaling support. Most evidence in PMOS and insulin resistance. Favorable safety profile. Add D-chiro-inositol at 40:1 ratio for best results.
Chromium	200–1,00 mcg/day (200–400 mcg most commonly) · Chromium picolinate	Enhances insulin receptor sensitivity. Adjunct to other insulin-sensitizing strategies. Not a standalone primary intervention.
Magnesium (glycinate or malate)	300–400 mg/day elemental magnesium · Divided doses with meals—especially your evening meal	Direct cofactor in insulin receptor activation; deficiency is common in insulin-resistant individuals and almost always missed by standard serum testing. Request RBC magnesium—not serum—to assess status accurately. Also improves sleep quality and reduces inflammatory markers. Loose stools indicate dose is too high; reduce and titrate up.
Choline (alpha-GPC)	250–500 mg/day · Choline bitartrate · Or 300–600 mg/day	Required for liver VLDL synthesis—the mechanism by which

	alpha-GPC for improved bioavailability	the liver packages and exports accumulated fat. Deficiency is common in low-egg diets and significantly more prevalent in postmenopausal women, who lose the estrogen-driven internal synthesis pathway. Prioritize dietary sources (egg yolks, liver, shrimp, salmon); supplement when intake is consistently low.
TIER 2 — Promising Evidence		
Silymarin (Milk Thistle)	420–600 mg/day · Phospholipid complex form (Siliphos/Phytosome) for best absorption	Liver cell membrane stabilizer, antioxidant, anti-fibrotic. Phospholipid complex absorbs 4–10× better than standard extract. Well-tolerated.
Curcumin	Follow product dosing · Enhanced-bioavailability form required (BCM-95, Meriva, Theracurmin, or CurcuWIN)	Anti-inflammatory (NF-kB), AMPK activator. Standard curcumin powder absorbs poorly—enhanced form is essential. Pairs well with berberine.

Green Tea Extract (EGCG)	400–800 mg/day · Standardized to EGCG content	Antioxidant, AMPK activator, liver fat reduction. Do not exceed 800 mg/day—rare hepatotoxicity reported at high doses. Better as brewed green tea for most.
Resveratrol	150–1,000 mg/day · Take with fat-containing meal	SIRT1 and AMPK activator. More consistent results in people with significant insulin resistance. Take with piperine or fat for improved absorption.
Artichoke Leaf Extract	600–1,800 mg/day · Standardized for cynarin	Supports bile flow and cholesterol metabolism. Best for those with elevated LDL, sluggish digestion, or impaired bile flow alongside MASLD.
Cinnamon Bark Extract	1–3 g/day · Ceylon cinnamon preferred over cassia	Modest insulin-sensitizing effect. Ceylon form avoids coumarin hepatotoxicity risk at supplemental doses. Reasonable low-cost adjunct.
N-Acetyl Cysteine (NAC)	600–1,800 mg/day · Divided into 2–3 doses daily	Replenishes hepatic glutathione—the liver's primary endogenous

		antioxidant—directly reducing the oxidative stress that drives progression from steatosis to MASH and fibrosis. Most relevant for those with elevated liver enzymes, confirmed steatohepatitis, or regular acetaminophen use (which depletes glutathione). Use with caution alongside nitrates or anticoagulants.
CoQ10 (ubiquinol)	100–300 mg/day · Ubiquinol form—significantly more bioavailable than ubiquinone, especially in adults over 40 · Take with a fat-containing meal	Supports mitochondrial fat oxidation and provides antioxidant protection in hepatic tissue. Most relevant for people on statin medications, which significantly deplete CoQ10 as a drug mechanism side effect. Also appropriate for those with persistent metabolic fatigue or suboptimal response to other interventions.
TUDCA (Tauroursodeoxy-cholic Acid)	500–1,750 mg/day · Divided doses	Reduces endoplasmic reticulum (ER) stress—a specific liver cell injury

		mechanism not addressed by other supplements in this table—and supports bile flow. Most relevant for those with confirmed steatohepatitis, markedly elevated liver enzymes, or incomplete response to standard supplement protocols. Consult physician before use if you have advanced liver disease, gallstones, or take bile acid sequestrants.
Quercetin	500–1,000 mg/day · Phytosome form or pair with vitamin C for improved absorption	Induces hepatic autophagy—the liver's self-clearing process for removing accumulated fat and damaged organelles—alongside NF-kB anti-inflammatory and antioxidant effects. Found in onions, capers, and apples; supplement for therapeutic doses. May mildly enhance anticoagulant effects at higher doses—monitor if taking blood thinners.

GUT HEALTH		
Multi-Strain Probiotic	10–50 billion CFU/day · Guaranteed potency through expiration · 5+ strains	Foundational daily supplement for most people. Key strains: *L. rhamnosus*, *L. acidophilus*, *B. longum*, *B. breve*. Use for minimum 8–12 weeks continuously. Pair with dietary fiber.
HORMONAL SUPPORT — Men		
Fenugreek (Fenutrax)	500–600 mg/day · Standardized to 50% saponins	Modest testosterone support, aromatase inhibition. Also improves insulin sensitivity. Double benefit for men with MASLD.
Tongkat Ali (LJ100)	200–400 mg/day · LJ100 extract	Improves free testosterone, reduces SHBG, supports body composition. Use clinically studied LJ100 form.
Ashwagandha (KSM-66)	300–600 mg/day · KSM-66 or Sensoril extract	Lowers cortisol, improves body composition, modest testosterone support. Best for men under chronic stress.
Shilajit	500 mg/day	Increases total and free testosterone and DHEA levels.

Tesnor (Cocoa bean and pomegranate peel extract)	200–400 mg	Increases total and free testosterone, boosts mood, enhances muscle strength, and reduces fatigue.
DIM (Diindolylmethane)	100–200 mg/day	Aromatase inhibition and estrogen metabolism support. Reduces estrogen dominance driven by visceral fat aromatization.
Calcium D-Glucarate	500–1,500 mg/day in divided doses	Supports estrogen clearance.
Supportive Nutrients	15–50 mg/day elemental Zinc (chelated form) · 400 mg magnesium (glycinate or malate form) · 10 mg vitamin B6 · vitamin D *Note: standard serum magnesium is an unreliable indicator of status — RBC magnesium is the appropriate test if assessing deficiency.*	Cofactors for testosterone production and hormone balance.
HORMONAL SUPPORT — Women		
DIM (Diindolylmethane)	100–300 mg/day	Shifts estrogen metabolism toward the 2-OH protective pathway. Most relevant for premenopausal estrogen dominance.

Calcium D-Glucarate	500–1,000 mg/day	Inhibits beta-glucuronidase to improve estrogen clearance. Use alongside DIM for comprehensive estrogen metabolism support.
Vitex / Chaste Tree (Ze 440)	Standardized (Ze 440 and Agnucaston): 20–40 mg/day · Dried fruit extract: 100–200 mg/day	Supports progesterone relative to estrogen in luteal phase. Best for PMS, irregular cycles, and progesterone insufficiency.
FenuSMART (*Trigonella foenum-graecum*; standardized to ≥10% protodioscin, ≥30% total saponins, trigonelline)	500–600 mg/day with food; Allow 4–8 weeks for measurable response	Protodioscin → DHEA precursor → supports endogenous estrogen & testosterone production. Trigonelline supports insulin signaling and androgen modulation. Avoid in pregnancy. Use caution with hormone-sensitive conditions. Consult physician if on HRT or with hormone-sensitive cancer history.
Ashwagandha (KSM-66)	300–600 mg/day	Cortisol reduction, thyroid support, perimenopausal hormonal balance.

Rhaptontic Rhubarb (*Rheum rhaponticum* root extract; ERr 731)	4 mg ERr 731 daily; take consistently for at least 8–12 weeks	Stilbene phytoestrogens (rhaponticin, desoxyrhaponticin) act as natural SERMs—selective estrogen receptor modulators. Reduces hot flash frequency/intensity 70–73% in RCTs. Does NOT stimulate breast or uterine tissue (confirmed by imaging). Supports bone metabolism markers and favorable cardiovascular markers. Relevant for post-menopausal MASLD progression.
Red MACA (gelatinized)	1.5–3.5 g	Promotes hormone balance and estrogen regulation.
Black Cohosh	20–80 mg/day	Reduces vasomotor symptoms associated with peri- to post-menopause.
Supportive Nutrients	400 mg magnesium (glycinate or malate form) · vitamin D · 2–4 g EPA/DHA *Note: standard serum magnesium is an unreliable indicator of status — RBC magnesium is the appropriate test if assessing deficiency.*	Cofactors for female hormone production and balance.

THYROID SUPPORT		
Selenium (Selenomethionine)	200 mcg/day	Essential for T4→T3 conversion and thyroid antioxidant protection. Reduces thyroid antibodies in Hashimoto's. Most evidence-supported thyroid supplement available.
Desiccated Organ Extracts (Thyroid and Liver)	As instructed on the product label	Supports thyroid and liver function.

Minimum viable protocol for most people with MASLD: Vitamin D3 (optimized to 40–80 ng/mL by testing) + Omega-3 fatty acids (2–4 g EPA/DHA daily) + Magnesium + Berberine (900–1,500 mg/day with meals) or Myo-Inositol (2–4 g/day) if insulin resistance is a primary concern + Multi-strain probiotic (daily, ongoing). These five address the most central metabolic and gut-liver axis mechanisms of fatty liver disease through distinct, well-documented pathways.

APPENDIX D

Lab Markers and How to Track Progress

Standard laboratory reference ranges are designed to capture the middle 95 percent of the general population—which, in a population where one in four adults has metabolic dysfunction, sets the bar too low for identifying early risk or optimizing health. The optimal target ranges in this appendix are based on expert clinical recommendations, population studies, and evidence from the MASLD literature specifically, not merely on avoiding clinical disease.

How to use this table: Bring it to your appointment, ask for the specific tests listed, and request a copy of your results. Track your values over time—improvement trends matter more than any single data point. A fasting insulin that has dropped from 18 to 9 μIU/mL over six months of lifestyle change is a profound metabolic win, even if 9 μIU/mL is still above the optimal target.

Marker	Standard Lab Range	Optimal Target Range	What It Tells You
LIVER ENZYMES			
ALT (Alanine aminotransferase)	<40 U/L (M) <31 U/L (F)	**< 20 U/L** Lower is better. Values at the upper end of 'normal' are associated with increased	Most sensitive liver enzyme for fatty liver. Elevated by hepatocyte stress and damage. Serial

		cardiovascular risk.	trending over time is as important as a single value.
AST (Aspartate aminotransferase)	<40 U/L	**< 20 U/L** AST:ALT ratio >2 may suggest alcohol-related rather than metabolic cause.	Often elevated alongside ALT. Used with ALT ratio to characterize liver involvement and rule out other etiologies.
GGT (Gamma-glutamyl transferase)	<65 U/L (M) <45 U/L (F)	**< 20 U/L (M) < 15 U/L (F)** One of the most sensitive early markers of liver metabolic stress.	Highly sensitive to fatty liver and alcohol. Often the first enzyme to rise. Elevated GGT is independently associated with cardiovascular risk.
Alkaline Phosphatase (ALP)	44–147 U/L	**Within lower half of lab range**	Less specific for MASLD but elevated in bile duct obstruction or advanced disease. Context-dependent interpretation.
INSULIN RESISTANCE & BLOOD SUGAR			
Fasting Glucose	70–99 mg/dL (normal) 100–125 mg/dL (prediabetes)	**70–85 mg/dL** Values at the upper end of "normal" often reflect early insulin resistance.	Blood sugar between meals. Values above 85 mg/dL when fasting consistently may indicate early metabolic dysfunction even within the 'normal' range.

Fasting Insulin	<25 μIU/mL	**2–6 μIU/mL** Not ordered routinely—ask specifically. Most powerful single test for insulin resistance.	The most underutilized and most informative metabolic test. Normal blood sugar with elevated fasting insulin is early, actionable insulin resistance.
HOMA-IR	<3.0 (calculated)	**< 1.5** Calculate: (Fasting Glucose × Fasting Insulin) ÷ 405	Composite insulin resistance score. Values above 2.0 are clinically significant. Values above 1.5 in the context of fatty liver disease warrant action.
HbA1c	< 5.7% (normal) 5.7–6.4% (prediabetes)	**4.8–5.2%** Values at 5.3–5.6% often reflect early metabolic dysfunction despite falling within "normal."	3-month average blood sugar. Trends matter more than single values. Improvement from 5.8% to 5.4% is a meaningful metabolic win.
LIPID PANEL			
Triglycerides	< 150 mg/dL	**< 80–100 mg/dL** Triglycerides above 100 mg/dL in the context of MASLD suggest active *de novo* lipogenesis.	Directly reflects liver fat production from excess carbohydrates. One of the most responsive markers to dietary improvement—often normalizes within weeks of reducing sugar.

HDL Cholesterol	> 40 mg/dL (M) > 50 mg/dL (F)	**> 60 mg/dL** Higher is better. Values below 40 (M) or 50 (F) indicate metabolic syndrome. disease and MASLD severity.	Low HDL is a component of metabolic syndrome and strongly correlated with insulin resistance. Rises reliably with exercise and dietary improvement.
LDL Cholesterol	< 100 mg/dL (general) < 70 mg/dL (high CV risk)	**Context-dependent** Particle size and number (LDL-P, ApoB) are more informative than LDL alone.	Standard LDL can be misleading in MASLD—small dense LDL particles are more atherogenic than large buoyant particles at the same LDL value. Request ApoB if available.
Triglyceride:HDL Ratio	< 3.5 (calculated)	mg/dL units (USA): **< 1.5** ideal · **1.5–2.0 caution** · **> 2.0** elevated risk · Ratio **> 3.0** strongly predicts insulin resistance and small dense LDL pattern; mmol/L units (Canada/UK/ Australia): < **0.5** ideal · **0.5–1.1** caution.	One of the most practically useful cardiovascular and insulin resistance markers. Divide your triglycerides by your HDL. Should trend down as metabolic health improves.

		MASLD-specific thresholds (mmol/L): > 0.54 is associated with measurable liver fat accumulation. > 0.73 is an emerging diagnostics threshold for MASLD in recent research. In mg/dL these correspond approximately to > 1.24 and > 1.68 respectively.	
INFLAMMATION & OTHER KEY MARKERS			
hsCRP (high-sensitivity C-reactive protein)	< 3.0 mg/L	**< 1.0 mg/L** Values 1–3 mg/L indicate intermediate cardiovascular risk. Values > 3 mg/L are high risk.	Sensitive systemic inflammation marker. Directly reflects the chronic low-grade inflammation central to MASH progression. Should improve with dietary quality, exercise, and visceral fat loss.
Ferritin	12–300 ng/mL (M) 12–150 ng/mL (F)	**50–100 ng/mL** Elevated ferritin (> 200 ng/mL) in MASLD is associated with greater fibrosis risk independent of iron overload.	Elevated in MASLD as an acute-phase inflammatory protein—not necessarily indicating iron overload. Serial

			monitoring helps distinguish inflammation-driven elevation from true hemochromatosis.
Platelet Count	150–400 K/µL	**Trend matters more than single value** A declining trend over years can precede clinical fibrosis diagnosis.	Platelets are produced with liver input and sequestered by an enlarging spleen in advancing fibrosis. A declining platelet count over serial measurements is a noninvasive fibrosis signal.
Vitamin D (25-OH)	20–50 ng/mL (standard sufficiency)	**40–80 ng/mL** For MASLD specifically: ≥ 44 ng/mL associated with ~60% lower disease odds.	Test before supplementing. Standard sufficiency thresholds are too low for liver health optimization. Retest 3 months after initiating supplementation to confirm dose adequacy.
Omega-3 Index (EPA+DHA % in RBCs)	>4% (low risk threshold varies by lab)	8–12% Values below 4% are associated with elevated cardiovascular and inflammatory risk. Values of 8–12% are associated with optimal liver fat reduction, lower	Measures actual EPA and DHA incorporation into red blood cell membranes—a direct tissue-level marker of omega-3 status, not dietary intake. Standard labs rarely include this; order through direct-to-

		inflammatory cytokines, and emerging fibrosis-protective effects.	consumer testing (OmegaQuant is the validated reference lab). Retest 3–4 months after adjusting dose.
Magnesium (RBC, not serum)	RBC Mg: 4.2–6.8 mg/dL	**5.6–6.8 mg/dL** (upper half of RBC reference range)—**Do not use serum magnesium to assess status.**	Approximately 99% of the body's magnesium is stored inside cells and bone—serum magnesium reflects only the tightly regulated extracellular fraction and remains normal until deficiency is severe. A normal serum magnesium result tells you almost nothing about true magnesium status. RBC magnesium is the appropriate functional test. Magnesium deficiency is common in insulin-resistant and metabolically unhealthy individuals and impairs glucose metabolism, blood pressure regulation, and sleep quality—all directly relevant to MASLD.

BODY COMPOSITION & PHYSICAL MARKERS			
Waist Circumference	< 40" (M) < 35" (F)—metabolic risk threshold	**< 35" (M) < 32" (F)** Measure at navel level, morning, standing naturally.	Most accessible proxy for visceral fat. More sensitive than BMI for MASLD risk and metabolic health tracking. Measure monthly—changes here often precede scale changes.
BMI	18.5–24.9 (standard normal)	**Not the primary target** Waist circumference + metabolic markers more informative than BMI alone for MASLD.	BMI does not distinguish visceral from subcutaneous fat and can be misleading in both directions. Use alongside waist circumference and metabolic markers, not instead of them.
FIB-4 Score	< 1.30 (low fibrosis risk) > 2.67 (high risk)—calculated	**< 1.30** Calculate: (Age × AST) ÷ (Platelets × √ALT)	Noninvasive fibrosis triage tool using routine labs. Free online calculators available. Scores between 1.30 and 2.67 warrant further evaluation (FibroScan or specialist referral).

Recommended testing schedule: Baseline (before beginning lifestyle program) → 3 months → 6 months → then annually if stable. More frequent monitoring is appropriate if medications are being adjusted, if disease stage is advanced, or if a new intervention has been introduced.

APPENDIX E

Questions to Ask Your Doctor

Most clinical appointments are short. Having specific, prepared questions ensures that the conversations most relevant to your liver health actually happen—rather than being displaced by administrative tasks or deferred to a future visit that may not occur. The following questions are organized by clinical context.

At Your Initial or Follow-Up Appointment

1. What is my current disease stage—do I have simple steatosis, MASH without fibrosis, or MASH with fibrosis? And at what stage?
2. Can you add fasting insulin to my next blood panel, in addition to fasting glucose? I would like to assess my HOMA-IR.
3. My triglyceride-to-HDL ratio is [X]—what does that suggest about my insulin resistance and cardiovascular risk?
4. Based on my FIB-4 score, do I need a FibroScan or specialist referral for further fibrosis staging?
5. What specific lifestyle changes would make the most meaningful difference for my specific situation and stage of disease?
6. Can you check my vitamin D level? I want to optimize it to 40–80 ng/mL for liver health, not just avoid deficiency.

If You Are Being Considered for Medication

1. What specific outcome is this medication expected to produce—liver fat reduction, fibrosis improvement, or something else—and over what timeframe?
2. What are the most serious potential side effects relevant to my health history and how will we monitor for them?
3. How does this medication interact with the lifestyle changes I am already making? Will I need to continue it indefinitely?
4. Are there lower-cost or better-established alternatives given my specific clinical picture?
5. If I optimize my lifestyle over the next six months, is there a realistic chance I can manage this without medication, or is pharmaceutical support clearly warranted at my current disease stage?

If Your Progress Has Stalled

1. My liver enzymes or metabolic markers have not improved despite consistent lifestyle effort—what additional investigations should we consider? Could thyroid dysfunction, sleep apnea, or hormonal imbalance be contributing?
2. Should I be screened for obstructive sleep apnea? I have [describe symptoms: snoring, unrefreshing sleep, morning headaches].
3. Is a referral to a hepatologist, endocrinologist, or registered dietitian appropriate at this stage?
4. I have a history of spending significant time in [region] / eating raw freshwater fish—should we rule out parasitic liver infection as a contributing factor?

For Ongoing Monitoring

1. Can we establish a monitoring schedule—lab recheck at three and six months, and FibroScan annually—so we are systematically tracking whether my strategy is working?

2. At what point would you consider my liver health sufficiently improved to reduce monitoring frequency?
3. Are there any new treatment options or clinical trials I should be aware of that might be relevant to my situation?

For Family Members and Screening

1. Given my diagnosis, should my close family members—particularly adult children—be screened for fatty liver disease or insulin resistance?
2. Are there specific genetic tests (PNPLA3, TM6SF2 variants) that would be informative for understanding my genetic risk and tailoring my management?
3. What symptoms should prompt me to seek earlier evaluation between scheduled appointments?

A Final Note on Advocating for Yourself

The most important conversation in your healthcare is the one where you tell your doctor, clearly and specifically, what your goals are. Most physicians are trained to respond to acute problems. Telling them that improving your liver health and metabolic function—not just managing symptoms—is a priorityshifts the entire orientation of your care. Bring your lab results. Ask for trends, not just single values. Request explanations in plain language. Follow up on unanswered questions. You are the most consistent presence in your own healthcare; use that position actively.

You now have the knowledge. The questions above give you the language. The rest is the conversation—and it is worth having.

References

[1] Le P, Tatar M, Dasarathy S, et al. Estimated Burden of Metabolic Dysfunction–Associated Steatotic Liver Disease in US Adults, 2020 to 2050. *Gastroenterol Hepatol.* 2025 Jan 17;8(1):e2454707.

[2] Mendex-Sanchez N, Brouwer WP, Lammert F, et al. Metabolic dysfunction associated fatty liver disease in healthy weight individuals. *Nature Link.* 2024 Jul;18:884-96.

[3] Yadav P, Quadri K, Kaudin R, et al. New approaches to the treatment of metabolic dysfunction-associated steatotic liver with natural products. *iLiver.* 2024 Dec;3(4):100131.

[4] GBD 2023 MASLD Collaborators. Global burden of metabolic dysfunction-associated steatotic liver disease, 1990–2023, and projections to 2050: a systematic analysis for the Global Burden of Disease Study 2023. *Gastroenterol Hepatol.* 2026 Apr 13. Online ahead of print.

[5] Gines P. Serra-Burriel M, Kamath PS. Metabolic Dysfunction–Associated Steatotic Liver Disease—The New Epidemic of Chronic Liver Disease. *Gastroenterol Hepatol.* 2025;8(6):e2516381.

[6] HCPLive; Brooks A. MASLD Prevalence Projected to Exceed 40% by 2050, Increasing Health System Burden. 2025 Jan 18. Accessed May 2, 2026 from: https://www.hcplive.com/view/masld-prevalence-projected-exceed-40-by-2050-increasing-health-system-burden.

[7] Wentworth BJ, Caldwell SH. Pearls and pitfalls in nonalcoholic fatty liver disease: tricky results are common. *Metab Target Organ Damage.* 2021 Jul 2;1(1):2.

[8] Dua A, Kumari R, Singh M, et al. Metabolic Dysfunction-Associated Steatotic Liver Disease (MASLD): the interplay of gut microbiome, insulin resistance, and diabetes. *Front Med (Lausanne).* 2025 Aug 14;12:1618275.

[9] Marjot T, Smith K, Westcott F, et al. Human MASLD is a diurnal disease driven by multisystem insulin resistance and reduced insulin availability at night. *Cell Metab.* 2026 Mar;38(3)::474-92.

[10] Marjot T, Smith K, Westcott F, et al. Human MASLD is a diurnal disease driven by multisystem insulin resistance and reduced insulin availability at night. *Cell Metab.* 2026 Mar;38(3)::474-92.

[11] Dhar D, Packer J, Michalopoulou S, et al. Assessing the evidence for health benefits of low-level weight loss: a systematic review. *Int J Obesity.* 2024 Nov;49:254-68.

[12] Dallio M, Sangineto M, Romeo M, et al. The influence of acute lifestyle changes on NAFLD evolution in a multicentre cohort: a matter of body composition. *Nutr Diabet.* 2024 May 27;14(33):2024.

[13] Stine JG, DiJoseph K, Pattison Z, et al. Exercise training is associated with treatment response in liver fat content by magnetic resonance imaging independent of clinically significant body weight loss in patients with

nonalcoholic fatty liver disease: a systematic review and meta-analysis. *Am J Gastroenterol.* 2023;118(7):1204-1213.
[14] Schwarz JM, Noworolski SM, Erkin-Cakmak A, et al. Effects of dietary fructose restriction on liver fat, de novo lipogenesis, and insulin kinetics in children with obesity. *Gastroenterology.* 2017;153(3):743-752.
[15] Tasali E, Wroblewski K, Kahn E, Loguinov A, Laumann AE, Riedel B. Effect of sleep extension on objectively assessed energy intake among adults with overweight in real-life settings: a randomized clinical trial. *JAMA Intern Med.* 2022;182(4):365-374.
[16] Daubenmier J, Kristeller J, Hecht FM, et al. Mindfulness intervention for stress eating to reduce cortisol and abdominal fat among overweight and obese women: an exploratory randomized controlled study. *JMB.* 2011;2011:1-13.
[17] Li Y, Yang P, Ye L, et al. Updated mechanisms of MASLD pathogenesis. *Nature Link.* 2024;23(117):2024.
[18] He Y, Chen Y, Qian S, et al. Immunopathogenic mechanisms and immunoregulatory therapies in MASLD. *Cell Molecular Immunol.* 2025;22:1159-77.
[19] Joslin Diabetes Center. High-fructose and high-fat diet damages liver mitochondria. *ScienceDaily.* 2019 Oct 1. Accessed May 4 at: www.sciencedaily.com/releases/2019/10/191001132712.htm.
[20] Yustisia I, Tandiari D, Cangara MH, et al. A high-fat, high-fructose diet induced hepatic steatosis, renal lesions, dyslipidemia, and hyperuricemia in non-obese rats. *Heliyon*, 2022;8(10):e10896.
[21] Jegatheesan P, De Bandt JP. Fructose and NAFLD: The multifaceted aspects of fructose metabolism. *Nutrients.* 2017;9(3):230.
[22] Schwarz JM, Noworolski SM, Erkin-Cakmak A, et al. Effects of dietary fructose restriction on liver fat, de novo lipogenesis, and insulin kinetics in children with obesity. *Gastroenterology.* 2017;153(3):743-752.
[23] Marjot T, Smith K, Westcott F, et al. Human MASLD is a diurnal disease driven by multisystem insulin resistance and reduced insulin availability at night. *Cell Metab.* 2026 Mar;38(3)::474-92.
[24] Gachon F, Bugianesi E, Castelnuovo G, et al. Potential bidirectional communication between the liver and the central circadian clock in MASLD. *NPJ Metab Health Dis.* 2025;3(1):15.
[25] Chen YJ, Yang BW, Gu ZC, et al. Interplay between circadian rhythms, gut microbiota, and MASLD: from mechanistic foundations to therapeutic opportunities. *Front Med.* 2026 Apr 14;13:2026.
[26] Harris WS. The Omega-6/Omega-3 ratio and cardiovascular disease: time for a more nuanced approach. *Clin Chem.* 2018;64(1):130-140.
[27] Merz KE, Thurmond DC. Role of Skeletal Muscle in Insulin Resistance and Glucose Uptake. *Compr Physiol.* 2020 Jul 8;10(3):785–809.
[28] Askari R, Rabani N, Marefati H, Azarnive MS, Pusceddu M, Migliaccio GM. Aerobic-resistance training with royal jelly supplementation has a

synergistic effect on paraoxonase 1 changes and liver function in women with MASLD. *Medicina*. 2025;61(2):349.
[29] Tasali E, Wroblewski K, Kahn E, Loguinov A, Laumann AE, Riedel B. Effect of sleep extension on objectively assessed energy intake among adults with overweight in real-life settings: a randomized clinical trial. *JAMA Intern Med*. 2022;182(4):365-374.
[30] Donga E, van Dijk M, van Dijk JG, et al. A single night of partial sleep deprivation induces insulin resistance in multiple metabolic pathways in healthy subjects. *J Clin Endocrinol Metab*. 2010;95(6):2963-2968.
[31] Xie L, Kang H, Xu Q, et al. Sleep drives metabolite clearance from the adult brain. *Science*. 2013;342(6156):373-377.
[32] Buxton OM, Pavlova M, Reid EW, Wang W, Simonson DC, Adler GK. Sleep restriction for 1 week reduces insulin sensitivity in healthy men. *Diabetes*. 2010;59(9):2126-2133.
[33] Donga E, van Dijk M, van Dijk JG, et al. A single night of partial sleep deprivation induces insulin resistance in multiple metabolic pathways in healthy subjects. *J Clin Endocrinol* Metab. 2010;95(6):2963-2968.
[34] Spiegel K, Tasali E, Penev P, Van Cauter E. Brief communication: Sleep curtailment in healthy young men is associated with decreased leptin levels, elevated ghrelin levels, and increased hunger and appetite. *Ann Intern Med*. 2004;141(11):846-850.
[35] St-Onge MP, Roberts AL, Chen J, et al. Short sleep duration increases energy intake but does not change energy expenditure in normal-weight individuals. *Am J Clin Nutr*. 2011;94(2):410-416.
[36] Weng JP, Sun JL, Chang KT, et al. Long-term shift work and the risk of metabolic dysfunction-associated steatotic liver disease: a prospective cohort study of 280,000 participants. *J Hepatol*. 2024;80(4):512-524.
[37] Chellappa SL, Atance DJ, Blackwell T, et al. Nighttime eating is associated with higher insulin resistance and lower glucose tolerance: a randomized crossover trial. *Sci Adv*. 2022;8(40):eabn8550.
[38] Issa AA, Shoval Y, Pace F. Ethanol-Producing Micro-Organisms of Human Gut: A Biological Phenomenon or a Disease? 2025 Jul 14;4(3):36.
[39] Yuan J, Chen C, Cui J, et al. Fatty liver disease caused by high-alcohol-producing Klebsiella pneumoniae. *Cell Metab*. 2019;30(4):675-688.e7.
[40] Mbaye B, Borentain P, Wasfy RM, et al. Endogenous Ethanol and Triglyceride Production by Gut Pichia kudriavzevii, Candida albicans and Candida glabrata Yeasts in Non-Alcoholic Steatohepatitis. *Cells*. 2022 Oct 27;11(21):3390.
[41] Huang T, Ma Y. Advances in biosynthesis of higher alcohols in Escherichia coli. *World J Microbiol Biotechnol*. 2023 Mar 21;39(125):2023.
[42] Wasfy RM, Mbaye B, Borentain P, et al. Ethanol-Producing Enterocloster bolteae Is Enriched in Chronic Hepatitis B-Associated Gut Dysbiosis: A Case–Control Culturomics Study. *Microorganisms*. 2023 Sep 28;11(10):2437.

43 Meijnikman AS, Gerdes VE, Nieuwdorp M, et al. Evaluating the contribution of gut-derived ethanol to the development of metabolic dysfunction-associated steatotic liver disease. *Nat Med.* 2022;28(10):2100-2111.

44 Yuan J, Chen C, Cui J, et al. Fatty liver disease caused by high-alcohol-producing Klebsiella pneumoniae. *Cell Metab.* 2019;30(4):675-688.e7.

45 Magueresse-Battistoni BL, Laboronne E, Vidal H, et al. Endocrine disrupting chemicals in mixture and obesity, diabetes and related metabolic disorders. *World J Biol Chem.* 2017 May 26;8(2):108–119.

46 Alonso-Magdalena P. The hidden health effects of endocrine-disrupting chemicals. *Nat Rev Endocrinol.* 2026;20:70-71.

47 Chen Y, Wang Y, Cui Z, et al. Endocrine disrupting chemicals: A promoter of non-alcoholic fatty liver disease. *Front Public Health.* 2023 Mar 21;11:2023.

48 Mosca A, Manco M, Braghini MR, et al. Environment, Endocrine Disruptors, and Fatty Liver Disease Associated with Metabolic Dysfunction (MASLD). 2024 Jan 21;14(1):71.

49 Kyrou I, Tsigos C. Stress hormones: cortisol and aldosterone. In: Feingold KR, Anawalt B, Blackman MR, et al, eds. *Endotext.* MDText.com, Inc; 2020.

50 Geer EB, Islam J, Buettner C. Mechanisms of glucocorticoid-induced insulin resistance: focus on adipose tissue function and lipid metabolism. *Endocrinol Metab Clin North Am.* 2014;43(1):75-102.

51 Saeed S, Charytan C, Charytan DM, et al. Perceived stress and its association with liver enzymes and metabolic markers in metabolic dysfunction-associated steatotic liver disease. *J Clin Med.* 2023;12(14):4752.

52 Tarantino G, Caputi A. Juggling metabolic dysfunction-associated steatotic liver disease and psychological stress. *World J Gastroenterol.* 2024;30(5):435-442.

53 Romeo S, Kozlitina J, Xing C, et al. Genetic variation in PNPLA3 confers susceptibility to nonalcoholic fatty liver disease. *Nat Genet.* 2008;40(12):1461-1465.

54 Anstee QM, Seth D, Day CP. Genetic factors that affect the onset and progression of nonalcoholic fatty liver disease. *Gastroenterology.* 2016;150(8):1728-1744.e7.

55 Longo M, Meroni M, Paolini E, et al. TM6SF2/PNPLA3/MBOAT7 Loss-of-Function Genetic Variants Impact on NAFLD Development and Progression Both in Patients and in In Vitro Models. *Cell Mol Gastroenterol Hepatol.* 2022;13(3):759-788.

56 Younossi ZM, Zelber-Sagi S, Henry L, et al. Lifestyle interventions in nonalcoholic fatty liver disease. *Gastroenterol Helpatol.* 2023 Jul 4;20:708-22.

57 Browning JD, Baker JA, Rogers T, et al. Short-term weight loss and hepatic triglyceride reduction: evidence of a metabolic advantage with dietary carbohydrate restriction. *Am J Clin Nutr.* 2011;93(5):1048-1052

[58] Mambrini SP, Grillo A, Colosimo S, et al. Diet and physical exercise as key players to tackle MASLD through improvement of insulin resistance and metabolic flexibility. *Front Nutr*. 2024;11:1426551

[59] Goodyear LJ, Kahn BB. Exercise, glucose transport, and insulin sensitivity. *Annu Rev Med*. 1998;49:235-261.

[60] Richter EA, Hargreaves M. Exercise, GLUT4, and skeletal muscle glucose uptake. *Physiol Rev*. 2013;93(3):993-1017.

[61] Musso G, Cassader M, Rosina F, et al. Impact of current treatments on liver histology and metabolic risk in nonalcoholic steatohepatitis: a systematic review and meta-analysis of randomized trials. *Diabetologia*. 2012;55(4):885-904.

[62] Vilar-Gomez E, Martinez-Perez Y, Calzadilla-Bertot L, et al. Weight loss through lifestyle modification significantly reduces features of nonalcoholic steatohepatitis. *Gastroenterology*. 2015;149(2):367-378.e5.

[63] Innes JK, Calder PC. Omega-6 fatty acids and inflammation. *Prostaglandins Leukot Essent Fatty Acids*. 2018;132:41-48.

[64] Hanhineva K, Törrönen R, Bondia-Pons I, et al. Impact of dietary polyphenols on carbohydrate metabolism. *Int J Mol Sci*. 2010;11(4):1365-1402.

[65] Fontana L, Eagon JC, Trujillo ME, et al. Visceral fat adipokine secretion is associated with systemic inflammation in obese humans. *Diabetes*. 2007;56(4):1010-1013.

[66] Tilg H, Adolph TE, Trauner M. Gut–liver axis: pathophysiological concepts and clinical implications. *Nat Rev Gastroenterol Hepatol*. 2021;18(4):261-277.

[67] Lambert JE, Ramos-Roman MA, Valdez MJ, et al. Weight loss in MASLD restores the balance of liver fatty acid sources. *J Clin Invest*. 2025 May 1;135(9):e174233.

[68] Vilar-Gomez E, Martinez-Perez Y, Calzadilla-Bertot L, et al. Weight loss through lifestyle modification significantly reduces features of nonalcoholic steatohepatitis. *Gastroenterology*. 2015;149(2):367-378.e5.

[69] Sodhi M, Mansour R, Westermann C, Etminan M. Risk of gastrointestinal adverse events associated with glucagon-like peptide-1 receptor agonists for weight loss. *JAMA*. 2023;310(14):1543-1545.

[70] Wilding JPH, Batterham RL, Calanna S, et al; STEP 1 Study Group. Once-weekly semaglutide in adults with overweight or obesity. *N Engl J Med*. 2021;384(11):989-1002.

[71] Feldstein AE, Werneburg NW, Canbay A, et al. Free fatty acids promote hepatic lipotoxicity by stimulating TNF-alpha expression via a lysosomal pathway. *Hepatology*. 2004;40(1):185-194.

[72] Hibbeln JR, Nieminen LR, Blasbalg TL, Riggs JA, Lands WE. Healthy intakes of n-3 and n-6 fatty acids: estimations considering worldwide dietary patterns. *Am J Clin Nutr*. 2006;83(6 Suppl):1483S-1493S.

[73] Laurindo LF, Laurindo LF, Rodriguex VD, et al. Evaluating the effects of seed oils on lipid profile, inflammatory and oxidative markers, and glycemic control of diabetic and dyslipidemic patients: a systematic review of clinical studies. *Front Nutr*. 2025 Feb 7;12:1502815.
[74] Voon PT, Ng CM, Ng YT, et al. Health Effects of Various Edible Vegetable Oils: An Umbrella Review. *Adv Nutr*. 2024 Sep;15(9):100276.
[75] DiNicolantonio JJ, O'Kefe JF. Omega-6 vegetable oils as a driver of coronary heart disease: the oxidized linoleic acid hypothesis. *Open Heart*. 2018 Sep 26;5(2):e000898.
[76] Feldstein AE, Werneburg NW, Canbay A, et al. Free fatty acids promote hepatic lipotoxicity by stimulating TNF-alpha expression via a lysosomal pathway. *Hepatology*. 2004;40(1):185-194.
[77] Franz MJ. Protein: controversies ad libitum. *Diabetes Spectr*. 2000;13(3):132-141.
[78] Gannon MC, Nuttall FQ, Neil BJ, Westphal SA. The insulin and glucose responses to meals of glucose plus various proteins in type II diabetic subjects. *Metabolism*. 1988;37(11):1081-1088.
[79] Holt SH, Miller JC, Petocz P, Farmakalidis E. A satiety index of common foods. *Eur J Clin Nutr*. 1995;49(9):675-690.
[80] Leidy HJ, Clifton PM, Astrup A, et al. The role of protein in weight loss and maintenance. *Am J Clin Nutr*. 2015;101(6):1320S-1329S.
[81] Hernández-Alonso P, Bulló M, Salas-Salvadó J. Dietary protein, weight loss, and weight maintenance. *Annu Rev Nutr*. 2016;36:331-354.
[82] Salas-Salvadó J, Bulló M, Estruch R, et al. Prevention of type 2 diabetes with the Mediterranean diet: a randomized trial. *Ann Intern Med*. 2011;154(1):1-9.
[83] Finicelli M, Salle AD, Galderisi U, et al. The Mediterranean Diet: An Update of the Clinical Trials. *Nutrients*. 2022 Jul 19;14(14):2956.
[84] Delarue J. Mediterranean Diet and cardiovascular diseases: A 2024 update. *Cahiers de Nutrition et de Diététique*. 2025 Feb;60(1):e1-e5.
[85] Martin-Pelaez S, Fito M, Castaner O. Mediterranean Diet Effects on Type 2 Diabetes Prevention, Disease Progression, and Related Mechanisms. A Review. *Nutrients*. 2020 Jul 27;12(8):2236.
[86] Giacco A, Cioffi F, Silvestri E. Mediterranean Diet and Metabolic Syndrome. *Nutrients*. 2025 Jul 18;17(14):2364.
[87] Haley AP, Knight-Scott J, Caillaud M, et al. Low carbohydrate and low-calorie diets reduce liver fat and lower brain glutamate and myo-inositol levels in patients with Metabolic Dysfunction-Associated Steatotic Liver Disease (MASLD). *Metab Brain Dis*. 2025 May;40(5).
[88] Mardinoglu A, Wu H, Lim JS, et al. An integrated understanding of lipid metabolic pathways that can be harnessed for the treatment of steatohepatitis. *Cell Metab*. 2018;27(3):559-571.e5.

89 Cai S, Geng J, Li S, et al. Efficacy and safety of time-restricted eating in metabolic dysfunction-associated steatotic liver disease: a 16-week randomized controlled trial. *J Hepatol.* 2024;81(1):15-24.

90 Li H, Li T. Intermittent Fasting versus Continuous Energy Restriction in MASLD: A Systematic Review and Meta-analysis. *Front Nutr.* 2026 Mar. Online ahead of print.

91 Ma L, Li H, Hu J, et al. Indole Alleviates Diet-induced Hepatic Steatosis and Inflammation in a Manner Involving Myeloid Cell PFKFB3. *Hepatol.* 2020 Oct;72(4):1191-1203.

92 Fink A, Rufer CE, Grandois JL, et al. Dietary walnut oil modulates liver steatosis in the obese Zucker rat. *Eur J Nutr.* 2013 Aug 13;53:645-60.

93 Sangouni AA, Azarmi S, Fallahzadeh H, et al. Effects of garlic on liver enzymes: a systematic review and meta-analysis of randomized controlled trials. *Diabetol Metab Syndr.* 2020;12:115.

94 Wastyk HC, Fragiadakis GK, Perelman D, et al. Gut-microbiota-targeted diets modulate human immune status. *Cell.* 2021;184(16):4137-4153.e14.

95 Vallianou NG, Kounatidis D, Psallida S, et al. The Interplay Between Dietary Choline and Cardiometabolic Disorders: A Review of Current Evidence. *Nature Link.* 2024 Mar;13:152-65.

96 Babu AF, Csader S, Lok J, et al. Positive effects of exercise intervention without weight loss and dietary changes in NAFLD-related clinical parameters: a systematic review and meta-analysis. *Nutrients.* 2021;13(9):3135.

97 Orci LA, Gariani K, Oldani G, et al. Exercise-based interventions for nonalcoholic fatty liver disease: a meta-analysis and meta-regression. *J Clin Exp Hepatol.* 2016;6(4):263-273.

98 Magkos F, Patterson BW, Mohammed BS, et al. Increased very-low-density lipoprotein triglyceride secretion during prolonged moderate-intensity exercise in humans. *J Clin Endocrinol Metab.* 2007;92(2):617-622.

99 Horowitz JF, Klein S. Lipid metabolism during endurance exercise. *Am J Clin Nutr.* 2000;72(2 Suppl):558S-563S.

100 Zhang T, Liu Y, Yang Y, et al. The Effect and Mechanism of Regular Exercise on Improving Insulin Impedance: Based on the Perspective of Cellular and Molecular Levels. *Int J Mol Sci.* 2025;26(9):4199.

101 Paquin J, Tremblay R, Islam H, et al. Resistance training, skeletal muscle hypertrophy, and glucose homeostasis: how related are they? A Systematic review and Meta-analysis. *Appl Physiol Mutr Metab.* 2024 Aug 8;49(12):1622-35.

102 Liu CH, Zeng QM, Kim W, et al. Sarcopenia and MASLD: novel insights and the future. *Nature Rev Endocrinol.* 2026;22:139-52.

103 Langer HT, et al. Weight loss with GLP-1 medicines does not result in a disproportionate loss of muscle mass or function in obese mice and humans. *Cell Metab.* 2026;38(3):418-430.

[104] Wilding JPH, Batterham RL, Calanna S, et al. Once-weekly semaglutide in adults with overweight or obesity. *N Engl J Med.* 2021;384(11):989-1002.
[105] Pedersen BK, Febbraio MA. Muscles, exercise and obesity: skeletal muscle as a secretory organ. *Nat Rev Endocrinol.* 2012;8(8):457-465.
[106] Vissers D, Hens W, Taeymans J, et al. The effect of exercise on visceral adipose tissue in overweight adults: a systematic review and meta-analysis. *PLoS One.* 2013;8(2):e56415.
[107] Keating SE, Hackett DA, George J, Johnson NA. Exercise and non-alcoholic fatty liver disease: a systematic review and meta-analysis. *J Hepatol.* 2012;57(1):157-166.
[108] Bacchi E, Negri C, Targher G, et al. Both resistance training and aerobic training reduce hepatic fat content in type 2 diabetic subjects with nonalcoholic fatty liver disease: the RAED2 randomized trial. *Hepatology.* 2013;58(4):1287-1295. doi:10.1002/hep.26393.
[109] Wan Y, Su Z. The Impact of Resistance Exercise Training on Glycemic Control Among Adults with Type 2 Diabetes: A Systematic Review and Meta-Analysis of Randomized Controlled Trials. *Biological Red Nurs.* 2024 Apr;26(4).
[110] Hannan AL, Hing W, Climstein M, et al. The effect of high-intensity interval training versus moderate-intensity continuous training on liver fat: a systematic review and meta-analysis. *J Clin Endocrinol Metab.* 2022;107(3):862-881.
[111] LaForgia J, Withers RT, Gore CJ. Effects of exercise intensity and duration on the excess post-exercise oxygen consumption. *J Sports Sci.* 2006;24(12):1247-1264.
[112] Jenkins EM, Nairn LN, Skelly LE, et al. Brief intermittent exercise ("exercise snacks") improves cardiorespiratory fitness and metabolic health. *Sci Rep.* 2019;9:9115.
[113] Dunstan DW, Kingwell BA, Larsen R, et al. Breaking up prolonged sitting reduces postprandial glucose and insulin responses. *Diabetes Care.* 2012;35(5):976-983.
[114] Hashimoto K, Dora K, Murakami Y, et al. Positive impact of a 10-min walk immediately after glucose intake on postprandial glucose levels. *Sci Reports.* 2025;15:22662.
[115] Bellini A, Nicolo A, Bazzucchi I, et al. The Effects of Postprandial Walking on the Glucose Response after Meals with Different Characteristics. *Nutrients.* 2022;14(5):1080.
[116] Zhang X, Wongpipit W, Sun F, et al. Walking Initiated 20 Minutes before the Time of Individual Postprandial Glucose Peak Reduces the Glucose Response in Young Men with Overweight or Obesity: A Randomized Crossover Study. *J Nutr.* 2021 Apr;151(4):866-75.
[117] Moore JM, Salmons H, Vinoskey C, et al. One minute of stair climbing and descending reduces postprandial insulin and glucose with 3-min improving insulin resistance following a mixed meal in young adults: A

randomized controlled crossover trial. *J Exercise Sci Fitness*. 2024 Jul;22(3):266-70.
[118] Saint-Maurice PF, Troiano RP, Bassett DR Jr, et al. Association of daily step count and step intensity with mortality among US adults. *JAMA Netw Open*. 2020;3(9):e2017176.
[119] Stefan N, Häring HU, Hu FB, et al. Metabolically healthy obesity: epidemiology, mechanisms, and clinical implications. *Lancet Diabetes Endocrinol*. 2013;1(2):152-162.
[120] Rytka JS, Wueest S, Gasser NS, et al. The portal theory: visceral adipose tissue and hepatic insulin resistance. *Am J Physiol Endocrinol Metab*. 2011;301(6):E1035-E1042.
[121] Nielsen S, Guo Z, Johnson CM, Hensrud DD, Jensen MD. Splanchnic lipolysis in human obesity. *J Clin Invest*. 2004;113(11):1582-1588.
[122] Kershaw EE, Flier JS. Adipose tissue as an endocrine organ. *J Clin Endocrinol Metab*. 2004;89(6):2548-2556.
[123] Petersen MC, Shulman GI. Mechanisms of insulin action and insulin resistance. *Physiol Rev*. 2018;98(4):2133-2223.
[124] Chaston TB, Dixon JB, O'Brien PE. Changes in fat-free mass during weight loss: a systematic review. *Int J Obes (Lond)*. 2007;31(5):743-759.
[125] Lönnqvist F, Thörne A, Nilsell K, et al. A pathogenic role of visceral fat hormone expression in abnormal fatty acid metabolism in obesity. *J Clin Invest*. 1995;95(3):1109-1116.
[126] Andersen T, Gluud C, Franzmann MB, et al. Hepatic effects of dietary weight loss in morbidly obese patients. *Hepatology*. 1991;13(4):641-647.
[127] Stokes CS, Lammert F. Excess Body Weight and Gallstone Disease. *Visc Med*. 2021;37(4):254–260.
[128] Lassailly G, Caiazzo R, Ntandja-Wandji LC, et al. Bariatric surgery provides long-term resolution of nonalcoholic steatohepatitis and regression of fibrosis. *Gastroenterology*. 2020;159(4):1290-1301.e5.
[129] Anderson JW, Konz EC, Frederich RC, et al. Long-term weight-loss maintenance: a meta-analysis of US studies. *Am J Clin Nutr*. 2001 Nov;74(5):579-84.
[130] Aviram R, Manella G, Asher G. The liver by day and by night. *J Hepatol*. 2021 May;74(5):1240-42.
[131] McAuliffe KE, Wary MR, Pleas GV, et al. Sleep insufficiency and life expectancy at the state-county level in the United States, 2019–2025. *SLEEP Adv*. 2025 Dec;6(4):zpaf090.
[132] Buxton OM, Pavlova M, Reid EW, et al. Sleep Restriction for 1 Week Reduces Insulin Sensitivity in Healthy Men. *Diabetes*. 2010 Jun 28;59(9):2126-33.
[133] Broussard JL, Kilkus JM, Delebecque F, et al. Elevated ghrelin predicts food intake during experimental sleep restriction. *Obesity (Silver Spring)*. 2015 Oct 15;24(1):132–138.

[134] Mosavat M, Mirsanjari M, Arabiat D, et al. The Role of Sleep Curtailment on Leptin Levels in Obesity and Diabetes Mellitus. *Obes Facts*. 2021 Mar 23;14(2):214–221.

[135] Spaeth AM, Goel N, Dinges DF. Caloric and Macronutrient Intake and Meal Timing Responses to Repeated Sleep Restriction Exposures Separated by Varying Intervening Recovery Nights in Healthy Adults. *Nutrients*. 2020 Sep 3;12(9):2694.

[136] Dickinson DL, Kakosche N, Drummond SPA. The impact of insufficient sleep on dietary choices and physical activity behaviors: evidence from a randomized cross-over trial. *Sci Reports*. 2025;15(24513).

[137] St-Onge M, Roberts A, Chen J, et al. Short sleep duration increases energy intakes but does not change energy expenditure in normal-weight individuals. *Am J Clin Nutr*. 2011;94(2):410-416.

[138] Andreeva VA, Perez-Jimenez J, st-Onge MP. A Systematic Review of the Bidirectional Association Between Consumption of Ultra-processed Food and Sleep Parameters Among Adults. *Curr Obes Rep*. 2023 Jul 21;12(4):439–452.

[139] Muzur A, Pace-Schott EF, Hobson JA. The prefrontal cortex in sleep. *Trends Cogn Sci*. 2002;6(11):475-481.

[140] Takahashi JS. Molecular components of the mammalian circadian clock. *Hum Mol Genet*. 2006;15(suppl_2):R271-R277.

[141] Zhang R, Lahens NF, Ballance HI, Hughes ME, Hogenesch JB. A circadian gene expression atlas in mammals: implications for biology and medicine. *Proc Natl Acad Sci U S A*. 2014;111(45):16219-16224.

[142] D'ettorre G, Pellicani V, Greco M, et al. Metabolic syndrome in shift healthcare workers. *Med Lav*. 2019 Aug 26;110(4):285–292.

[143] Lee Y, Lee W. Shift work and non-alcoholic fatty liver disease in young, healthy workers. *Sci Reports*. 2024;14(19367).

[144] Scheer FA, Hilton MF, Mantzoros CS, Shea SA. Adverse metabolic and cardiovascular consequences of circadian misalignment. *Proc Natl Acad Sci U S A*. 2009;106(11):4453-4458.

[145] Saitmuratovna YA. THE METABOLIC PATHWAY OF CORTISOL IN CHRONIC STRESS: A SYSTEMATIC LITERATURE REVIEW. *EPRA Int H Multidisciplinary Res*. 2025 Sep;11(90:2455-3662.

[146] Martinez GJ, Kipp ZA, Lee WH, et al. Glucocorticoid resistance remodels liver lipids and prompts lipogenesis, eicosanoid, and inflammatory pathways. *Prostaglandins Other Lipid Mediators*. 2024 Aug;173:106840.

[147] Ullah A, Singla RK, Batool Z, et al. Pro- and anti-inflammatory cytokines are the game-changers in childhood obesity-associated metabolic disorders (diabetes and non-alcoholic fatty liver diseases). *Springer Nature Link*. 2024 May;25:783-803.

[148] Elwing JE, Lustman PJ, Wang HL, Clouse RE. Depression, anxiety, and nonalcoholic steatohepatitis: a new model of inflammation. *Hepatology*. 2006;44(1):174-180.

[149] Yu T, Zhou Y, Wu X, et al. Association Between Obstructive Sleep Apnea and Non-Alcoholic Fatty Liver Disease: Epidemiological Cross-Sectional Study and Mendelian Randomization Analysis. *Nat Sci Sleep*. 2025 Jun 17;17:1361–1376.
[150] Zhao ZW, Huang WS, Li L, et al. Association between sleep apnea and ultrasound-defined liver fibrosis: Results from NHANES 2017 to 2020. *Medicine (Baltimore)*. 2024 Apr 26;103(17):e37949.
[151] Amen S, Rasool B, Al Lami BS, et al. Obstructive Sleep Apnea and Cardiovascular Diseases: A Systematic Review and Meta-Analysis of Prospective Studies. *Cureus*. 2024 Oct 18;16(10):e71752.
[152] Channapragada TV, Brenner CR, Guruswamy K, et al. Does Continuous Positive Airway Pressure Improve Liver Outcomes in MASLD with Obstructive Sleep Apnea? A Systematic Review. *J Clin Med*. 2025 Dec 27;15(1):225.
[153] Inchingolo AD, Inchingolo AM, Ciocia C, et al. Efficacy of Mandibular Advancement Devices in the Treatment of Mild to Moderate Obstructive Sleep Apnea: A Systematic Review. *Int J Transl Med*. 2025;5(4):49.
[154] Kushner RF, Blatner DJ. Lifestyle change: dual-focused and multifaceted. *Med Clin North Am*. 2011;95(5):927-941.
[155] Khoury B, Sharma M, Rush SE, et al. Mindfulness-based stress reduction for healthy individuals: a meta-analysis. *J Psychosom Res*. 2015;78(6):519-528.
[156] Mazzali L, Albornoz S, de Medeiros G, et al. Effectiveness of a mindfulness-based intervention in the management of non-alcoholic fatty liver disease: a randomized controlled pilot study. *Eat Weight Disord*. 2022;27(4):1455-1463.
[157] Tincani G, Mazzali L, Albornoz S, et al. Mindfulness-based intervention in non-alcoholic fatty liver disease (NAFLD): a systematic review of the literature. *Health Psychol Rev*. 2021;15(4):564-582.
[158] Park BJ, Tsunetsugu Y, Kasetani T, et al. The physiological effects of Shinrin-yoku (taking in the forest atmosphere or forest bathing): evidence from field experiments in 24 forests across Japan. *Environ Health Prev Med*. 2009 May 2;15(1):18–26.
[159] Knauft K, Israil LZ, Zilioli S. The Endocrinology of Loneliness and Social Isolation. *Handbook Lonliness*. 2025 Nov:225-35.
[160] Holt-Lunstad J, Smith TB, Layton JB. Social relationships and mortality risk: a meta-analytic review. *PLoS Med*. 2010;7(7):e1000316.
[161] Ittermann T, Haring R, Wallaschofski H, et al. Inverse association between serum free thyroxine levels and hepatic steatosis: results from the Study of Health in Pomerania. *Thyroid*. 2012;22(6):568-574.
[162] Kasarinaite A, Sinton M. Sunders PT, et al. The Influence of Sex Hormones in Liver Function and Disease. *Cells*. 2023 Jun 11;12(12):1604.

[163] Hamamah S, Iatcu OC, Covasa M. Dietary Influences on Gut Microbiota and Their Role in Metabolic Dysfunction-Associated Steatotic Liver Disease (MASLD). *Nutrients*. 2025;17(1):143.
[164] Sender R, Fuchs S, Milo R. Revised Estimates for the Number of Human and Bacteria Cells in the Body. *PLoS Biol.* 2016 Aug 19;14(8):e1002533.
[165] Leviatan S, Shoer S, Rothschild D, et al. An expanded reference map of the human gut microbiome reveals hundreds of previously unknown species. *Nature Comun*. 2022;13(3863).
[166] Afzaal M, Saeed F, Shah YA, et al. Human gut microbiota in health and disease: Unveiling the relationship. *Front Microbiol.* 2022 Sep 25;13(2022).
[167] Chen H, Wang Y, Su W, et al. Therapeutic modulation of the gut-liver axis with faecalibacterium prausnitzii in metabolic dysfunction-associated steatohepatitis. *BMC Microbiol.* 2026;26(382).
[168] Asghari P, Ahmadi-Khorram M, Hatami A, et al. Therapeutic potential of Akkermansia muciniphila in non-alcoholic fatty liver disease: a systematic review. *BMC Gastroenterol.* 2025 Nov 19;25:822.
[169] Nadeau BA, Comjeevaram H. The gut microbiome and nonalcoholic fatty liver disease. *Clin Liver Dis (Hoboken).* 2017 Nov 30;10(5):116–119.
[170] Iruzubieta P, Medina JM, Fernandez-Lopez R, et al. A Role for Gut Microbiome Fermentative Pathways in Fatty Liver Disease Progression. *J Clin Med.* 2020 May 7;9(5):1369.
[171] Garcia-Mateo S, Rondinella D, Ponziana FR, et al. Gut microbiome and metabolic dysfunction-associated steatotic liver disease: Pathogenic role and potential for therapeutics. *Best Pract Res Clin Gastroenterol.* 2024 Sep;72:101924.
[172] Di Vincenzo F, Del Gaudio A, Petito V, et al. Gut microbiota, intestinal permeability, and systemic inflammation: a narrative review. *Intern Emerg Med.* 2023 Jul 28;19(2):275–293.
[173] Issa AA, Shoval Y, Pace F. Ethanol-Producing Micro-Organisms of Human Gut: A Biological Phenomenon or a Disease? *Appl Biosci.* 2025;4(3):36.
[174] Meijnikman AS, Nieuwdorp M. Schnabl B. Endogenous ethanol production in health and disease. *Natur Rev Gastroenterol Hepatol.* 2024;21:556-71.
[175] Bishehsari F, Magno E, Swanson G, et al. Alcohol and Gut-Derived Inflammation. *Alcohol Res*. 2017;38(2):163–171.
[176] Chen X, Zhang Z, Li H, et al. Endogenous ethanol produced by intestinal bacteria induces mitochondrial dysfunction in non-alcoholic fatty liver disease. *J Gastroenterol Hepatol. 2020* Mar 9;35(11).
[177] Meijnikman AS, Davids M, Herrema H, et al. Microbiome-derived ethanol in nonalcoholic fatty liver disease. *Nature Med.* 2022 Oct;28:2100-06.
[178] Qin X, Chen M, He B, et al. Role of short-chain fatty acids in non-alcoholic fatty liver disease and potential therapeutic targets. *Front microbiol.* 2025 Apr 2;16(2025).

[179] American Gut Project. Accessed May 4, 2026 at: https://microbeatlas.org/project?pid=ERP012803.
[180] Federico A, Dallio M, Masarone M, et al. The role of fiber in the treatment of non-alcoholic fatty liver disease: a systematic review. *Nutrients*. 2017;9(10):1152.
[181] Anderson JW, Baird P, Davis RH Jr, et al. Health benefits of dietary fiber. *Nutr Rev*. 2009;67(4):188-205.
[182] Hajiaghaalipour F, Akhlaghi M, Dehghan P. Effects of soluble fiber supplementation on liver enzymes and metabolic markers in patients with non-alcoholic fatty liver disease: a systematic review and meta-analysis of randomized controlled trials. *Complement Ther Med*. 2021;60:102754.
[183] Bird AR, Conlon MA, Christophersen CT, et al. Resistant starch, colorectal health, and genetic susceptibility to colorectal cancer. *Curr Colorectal Cancer Rep*. 2010;6(4):232-239.
[184] Ni Y, Qian L, Siliceo SL, et al. Resistant starch decreases intrahepatic triglycerides in patients with non-alcoholic fatty liver disease via gut microbiome alterations. *Cell Metab*. 2023;35(9):1530-1548.e8.
[185] Cani PD, Joly E, Horsmans Y, et al. Oligofructose promotes satiety in healthy humans: a randomized fixed-dose study. *Eur J Clin Nutr*. 2006;60(5):567-572.
[186] Wastyk HC, Fragiadakis GK, Perelman D, et al. Gut-microbiota-targeted diets modulate human immune status. *Cell*. 2021;184(16):4137-4153.e14.
[187] Hertzler SR, Clancy SM. Kefir improves lactose digestion and tolerance in adults with lactose maldigestion. *J Am Diet Assoc*. 2003;103(5):582-587.
[188] Sharpton SR, Maraj B, Harding-Theobald E, et al. Efficacy of probiotics, prebiotics, and synbiotics in nonalcoholic fatty liver disease: a systematic review and meta-analysis. *Am J Clin Nutr*. 2019;109(4):1111-1121.
[189] Kobyliak N, Abenavoli L, Mykhalchyshyn G, et al. A multi-strain probiotic "Symbiter" for prophylaxis and treatment of non-alcoholic fatty liver disease: a double-blind RT. *BMJ Open Gastroenterol*. 2018;5(1):e000213.
[190] Craven L, Rahman A, Nair Parvathy S, et al. Allogenic fecal microbiota transplantation in patients with nonalcoholic fatty liver disease: a randomized placebo-controlled trial. *Am J Gastroenterol*. 2020;115(12):1998-2007.
[191] Salminen S, Collado MC, Endo A, et al. The International Scientific Association for Probiotics and Prebiotics (ISAPP) consensus statement on the definition and scope of postbiotics. *Nat Rev Gastroenterol Hepatol*. 2021;18(9):649-667.
[192] Mattace Raso G, Simeoli R, Russo R, et al. Effects of sodium butyrate on non-alcoholic fatty liver disease in mice: a potential role of the SIRT1/AMPK pathway. *Eur J Nutr*. 2013;52(2):501-509.
[193] Gan L, Feng Y, Du B, et al. Bacteriophage targeting microbiota alleviates non-alcoholic fatty liver disease induced by high alcohol-producing Klebsiella pneumoniae. *Nature Commun*. 2023;14(3215).

[194] Hsu C, Duan Y, Fouts DE, et al. Intestinal virome and therapeutic potential of bacteriophages in liver disease. *J Hepatol.* 2021 Aug 24;75(6):1465–1475.
[195] Berry SE, Valdes AM, Drew DA, et al. Human postprandial responses to food and potential for personalized nutrition. *Nat Med.* 2020;26(6):964-973.
[196] Jump DB, Depner CM, Tripathy S. Omega-3 fatty acid supplementation and non-alcoholic fatty liver disease. *Metabolism.* 2012;61(10):1344-1356.
[197] Menni C, Zierer J, Pallister T, et al. Omega-3 fatty acids correlate with gut microbiome diversity and production of N-carbamylglutamate in middle-aged and elderly women. *Sci Rep.* 2017;7(1):11079.
[198] Yan JH, Guan BJ, Gao HY, et al. Omega-3 polyunsaturated fatty acid supplementation and non-alcoholic fatty liver disease: a meta-analysis of randomized controlled trials. *Medicine (Baltimore).* 2018;97(37):e12271.
[199] Musa-Veloso K, Vendittie C, Lee HY, et al. Systematic review and meta-analysis of controlled intervention studies on the effectiveness of long-chain omega-3 fatty acids in patients with nonalcoholic fatty liver disease. *Nutr Rev.* 2018 Aug;76(8):581-602.
[200] Lee CH, Fu Y, Yang SJ, et al. Effects of Omega-3 Polyunsaturated Fatty Acid Supplementation on Non-Alcoholic Fatty Liver: A Systematic Review and Meta-Analysis. 2020 Sep;12(9):2769.
[201] Sanyal AJ, Chalasani N, Kowdley KV, et al. Pioglitazone, vitamin E, or placebo for nonalcoholic steatohepatitis. *N Engl J Med.* 2010;362(18):1675-1685
[202] Miller ER 3rd, Pastor-Barriuso R, Dalal D, et al. Meta-analysis: high-dosage vitamin E supplementation may increase all-cause mortality. *Ann Intern Med.* 2005;142(1):37-46.
[203] Klein EA, Thompson IM Jr, Tangen CM, et al. Vitamin E and the risk of prostate cancer: the Selenium and Vitamin E Cancer Prevention Trial (SELECT). *JAMA.* 2011;306(14):1549-1556.
[204] Chen L, Zhang H, Miller S, et al. Hepatic microRNA-93 drives the pathogenesis of MASLD by targeting the SIRT1/AMPK signaling axis. *Metabolism.* 2025;162:155892.
[205] Kamanna VS, Ganji SH, Kashyap ML. The mechanism and mitigation of niacin-induced flushing. *Int J Clin Pract.* 2009;63(9):1369-1377.
[206] Nazari A, Ghotbabadi ZR, Kazemi KS, et al. The Effect of Berberine Supplementation on Glycemic Control and Inflammatory Biomarkers in Metabolic Disorders: An Umbrella Meta-analysis of Randomized Controlled Trials. *Clin Therapeutics.* 2024 Feb;46(2):e64-e72.
[207] Ji J, Li Y, Xu T, et al. Protective effects of berberine on MASLD: regulation of glucose and lipid metabolism through PI3K/Akt and STING pathways. *Nature Link.* 2025 Mar;398:12405-20.
[208] Liang Y, Xu X, Yin M, et al. Effects of berberine on blood glucose in patients with type 2 diabetes mellitus: a systematic review and meta-analysis

of randomized controlled trials. *Evid Based Complement Alternat Med.* 2019;2019:1431474.
[209] Yin J, Xing H, Ye J. Efficacy of berberine in patients with type 2 diabetes mellitus. *Metabolism*. 2008;57(5):712-717.
[210] Zhang LS, Wang DX, Zhang JH, et al. Berberine alleviates metabolic syndrome by modulating gut microbiota and increasing *Akkermansia muciniphila* abundance. *Theranostics*. 2019;9(24):7360-7376.
[211] Eliades M, Spyrou E, Agopian N, et al. Meta-analysis: vitamin D and non-alcoholic fatty liver disease. *Aliment Pharmacol Ther*. 2013;38(3):246-254.
[212] Thompson RL, Vance KJ, Morales AJ, et al. Serum 25-hydroxyvitamin D thresholds and the risk of metabolic dysfunction-associated steatotic liver disease: a cross-sectional analysis of the 2024-2025 cohort. *Nutrients*. 2026;18(5):1124.
[213] Unfer V, Facchinetti F, Orrù B, Giordani B, Nestler J. Myo-inositol effects in women with PCOS: a meta-analysis of randomized controlled trials. *Endocr Connect*. 2017;6(8):647-658.
[214] Minambres I, Cuixart G, Goncalves A, et al. Effects of inositol on glucose homeostasis: Systematic review and meta-analysis of randomized controlled trials. *Clin Nutr*. 2019 Jun;38(3):1146-52.
[215] Nordio M, Proietti E. The combined therapy with myo-inositol and D-chiro-inositol (40:1) is more effective than myo-inositol therapy alone in achieving ovulation in PCOS patients. *Eur Rev Med Pharmacol Sci.* 2012;16(5):575-581.
[216] Vincent JB. The biochemistry of chromium. *Angew Chem Int Ed Engl.* 2004;43(39):5126-5133.
[217] Suksomboon N, Poolsup N, Yuwanakorn A. Systematic review and meta-analysis of the efficacy and safety of chromium supplementation in diabetes. *J Clin Pharm Ther*. 2014;39(3):292-306.
[218] Wan S, He J, Simoes EJ, et al. Chromium Supplementation to Reduce Cardiometabolic Risk Factors:
A Novel Dose-Response Meta-Analysis of Randomized Clinical Trials. *JACC Adv*. 2023 Nov 23;2(10):100729.
[219] Al Alawi AM, Majoni SW, Faljammar H. Magnesium and Human Health: Perspectives and Research Directions. *Int J Endocrinol.* 2018 Apr 16;2018:9041694.
[220] Pelczynska M, Moszak M, Bogdanski P. The Role of Magnesium in the Pathogenesis of Metabolic Disorders. *Nutrients*. 2022;14(9):1714.
[221] Basit A, Kumar S, Ahmed H, et al. Impact of oral magnesium supplementation on glycemic and cardiometabolic outcomes in prediabetic adults: a systematic review and meta-analysis. 2026;25(45):(2026).
[222] Xu L, Li X, Wang X, et al. Effects of magnesium supplementation on improving hyperglycemia, hypercholesterolemia, and hypertension in type 2 diabetes: A pooled analysis of 24 randomized controlled trials. *Front Nutr*. 2023 Jan 17;9:(2022).

[223] Veronese N, Dominguez LJ, Pizzol D, et al. Oral magnesium supplementation for glycemic control in inflammation: Is it time? *Nutrients*. 2019;11(12):2988.
[224] Mariforta UM, Millet O, Lu SC, et al. Dysfunctional VLDL metabolism in MASLD. *Npj Metabol Health Dis*. 2024;2(16).
[225] Resseguie ME, da Costa KA, Galanko JA, et al. Aberrant Estrogen Regulation of PEMT Results in Choline Deficiency-associated Liver Dysfunction. *J Biol Chem*. 2010 Nov 8;286(2):1649–1658.
[226] Li S, Zhang G, Li X, et al. Choline Deficiency Drives the Inflammation–Fibrosis Cascade: A Spatiotemporal Atlas of Hepatic Injury from Weeks 6 to 10. 2026 Jan;15(1):110.
[227] Li S, Zhang G, Li X, et al. Choline Deficiency Drives the Inflammation–Fibrosis Cascade: A Spatiotemporal Atlas of Hepatic Injury from Weeks 6 to 10. 2026 Jan;15(1):110.
[228] Taesuwan S, Kouvari M, McKune AJ, et al. Total choline intake, liver fibrosis and the progression of metabolic dysfunction-associated steatotic liver disease: Results from 2017 to 2020 NHANES. *Maturitas*. 2025 Jan;191:108150.
[229] Trappoliere M, Caligiuri A, Schmid M, et al. Silybin, a component of silymarin, exerts anti-inflammatory and anti-fibrotic effects on human hepatic stellate cells. *J Hepatol*. 2009;50(6):1102-1111.
[230] Zhong S, Fan Y, Yan Q, et al. The therapeutic effect of silymarin in the treatment of nonalcoholic fatty liver disease: a meta-analysis (PRISMA) of randomized control trials. *Medicine (Baltimore)*. 2017;96(49):e9039.
[231] Morazzoni P, Magistretti MJ, Giachetti C, et al. Comparative bioavailability of Silipide, a new flavanolignan complex, in rats. *Eur J Drug Metab Pharmacokinet*. 1992;17(1):39-44.
[232] Zhu B, Ding Z, Rong X, et al. Silybin Cocrystals with Improved Solubility and Bioavailability. *Pharmaceuticals (Basel)*. 2025 Jan 13;18(1):90.
[233] Aggarwal BB, Yuan W, Li S, et al. Curcumin-free turmeric exhibits anti-inflammatory and anticancer activities: Identification of novel components of turmeric. *Molecular Nutrition & Food Research*. 2013;57(9):1529-1542.
[234] Sun D, Wang J, Li J, et al. Advances and Perspectives in Curcumin Regulation of Systemic Metabolism: A Focus on Multi-Organ Mechanisms. *Antioxidants*. 2026;15(1):109.
[235] Scazzocchio B, Minghetti L, D'Archivio M. Interaction between Gut Microbiota and Curcumin: A New Key of Understanding for the Health Effects of Curcumin. *Nutrients*. 2020 Aug 19;12(9):2499.
[236] Jalali M, Mahmoodi M, Moosavian SP, et al. The effects of curcumin supplementation on liver function, metabolic profile and body composition in patients with non-alcoholic fatty liver disease: a systematic review and meta-analysis of randomized controlled trials. *Complement Ther Med*. 2020;48:102283.

[237] Goodarzi R, Sabzchi-Zehni M, Alizadeh M. The effect of curcumin supplementation on liver enzymes in patients with non-alcoholic fatty liver disease: a systematic review and meta-analysis of randomized controlled trials. *Complement Ther Med*. 2019;44:230-237.
[238] Hegde M, Girisa S, BharathwajChetty B, et al. Curcumin Formulations for Better Bioavailability: What We Learned from Clinical Trials Thus Far? *ACS Omega*. 2023 Mar 13;8(12):10713–10746.
[239] Cicero AFG, Fogacci F, Hernandez AV, et al. Efficacy and safety of berberine and curcumin synergistic formulations in metabolic syndrome: A 2025 meta-analysis. *Nutrients*. 2025;17(3):812.
[240] Zhang Y, Yin R, Lang J, et al. Epigallocatechin-3-gallate ameliorates hepatic damages by relieve FGF21 resistance and promotion of FGF21–AMPK pathway in mice fed a high fat diet. *Diabetol Metab Syndr*. 2022 Apr 13;14:53.
[241] Yang J, Chen W, Chen J, et al. Tea Polyphenol Epigallocatechin Gallate and the Gut–Health Axis: Unraveling Structural Characteristics, Metabolic Pathways, and Systemic Benefits. *Adv Nutr*. 2025 Dec;16(12):100545.
[242] Mansoori A, Hosseini SA, Zilaee M, Hormoznejad R, et al. Effect of green tea consumption on liver enzymes in patients with non-alcoholic fatty liver disease: A systematic review and meta-analysis of randomized controlled trials. *Complement Ther Med*. 2018;40:1-7.
[243] Saleh IG, Ali Z, Abe N, et al. Possible hepatocellular toxicity of EGCG under the influence of an inflammagen. *J Appl Biomed*. 2014 Nov;12(4):291-9.
[244] Baur JA, Pearson KJ, Price NL, et al. Resveratrol improves health and survival of mice on a high-calorie diet. *Nature*. 2006;444(7117):337-342.
[245] Kantartzis K, Fritsche L, Bombrich M, et al. Effects of resveratrol supplementation on liver fat content in overweight and obese subjects: a randomized, double-blind, placebo-controlled trial. *Diabetes Care*. 2014;37(7):1-3.
[246] Speroni E, Cervellati R, Govoni P, et al. Efficacy of different *Cynara scolymus* preparations on liver complaints. *J Ethnopharmacol*. 2003;86(2-3):203-211.
[247] Amini MR, Sheikhhossein F, Talebyan A, et al. Effects of Artichoke Supplementation on Liver Enzymes: A Systematic Review and Meta-Analysis of Randomized Controlled Trials. *Clin Nutr Res*. 2022 Jul 25;11(3):228–239.
[248] Zarezadeh M, Musazadeh V, Foroumandi E, et al. The effect of cinnamon supplementation on glycemic control in patients with type 2 diabetes or with polycystic ovary syndrome: an umbrella meta-analysis on interventional meta-analyses. *Diabetol Metab Syndr*. 2023 Jun 15;15:127.
[249] Gou H, Zhong L, Wei Q, et al. The effects of cinnamon on patients with metabolic diseases: an umbrella review of meta-analyses of randomized controlled trials. *Front Nutr*. 2025 Nov;12:2025.

[250] Khan A, Safdar M, Ali Khan MM, et al. Cinnamon improves glucose and lipids of people with type 2 diabetes. *Diabetes Care*. 2003;26(12):3215-3218.
[251] Sinaeinejad M, Karimi M, Razavizadeh M, et al. Efficacy of N-Acetylcysteine on Liver Function and Metabolic Profiles in Patients with Metabolic Dysfunction-Associated Steatotic Liver Disease (MASLD): A Double-Blind, Randomized Controlled Trial. *Addict Health*. 2025 Jan:17:1667.
[252] Vrentzos E, Ikonomidis I, Pavlidis G, et al. Six-month supplementation with high dose coenzyme Q10 improves liver steatosis, endothelial, vascular and myocardial function in patients with metabolic-dysfunction associated steatotic liver disease: a randomized double-blind, placebo-controlled trial. *Cardiovascular Diabetol*. 2024 Jul;23(245):(2024).
[253] Ardekani A, Tabrizi R, Maleki E, et al. Effects of coenzyme Q10 supplementation on lipid profiles and liver enzymes of nonalcoholic fatty liver disease (NAFLD) patients: A systematic review and meta-analysis of randomized controlled trials. *Food Sci Nutr*. 2023 Mar 13;11(6):2580-2588.
[254] Zhang Y, Qu P, Ma X, et al. Tauroursodeoxycholic acid (TUDCA) alleviates endoplasmic reticulum stress of nuclear donor cells under serum starvation. *PLOS One*. 2018 May;13(5):e0196785.
[255] Kars M, Yang L, Gregor MF, et al. Tauroursodeoxycholic Acid May Improve Liver and Muscle but Not Adipose Tissue Insulin Sensitivity in Obese Men and Women. *Diabetes*. 2010 Jun 3;59(8):1899–1905.
[256] Portincasa P, Palmieri V, Doronzo F, et al. Effect of tauroursodeoxycholic acid on serum liver enzymes and dyspeptic symptoms in patients with chronic active hepatitis. *Curr Ther Res*. 1993 May;53(5):521-32.
[257] Guo Z, Zhang J, Li M, et al. Mechanism of action of quercetin in regulating cellular autophagy in multiple organs of Goto-Kakizaki rats through the PI3K/Akt/mTOR pathway. *Front Med*. 2024 Aug 14;11:2024.
[258] Katsaros I, Sotiropoulou M, Vailas M, et al. Quercetin's Potential in MASLD: Investigating the Role of Autophagy and Key Molecular Pathways in Liver Steatosis and Inflammation. *Nutrients*. 2024 Nov 5;16(22):3789.
[259] Kin D, Kin S, Zhou T, et al. Effects of Quercetin on Metabolic Dysfunction-Associated Steatotic Liver Disease: A Systematic Review and Meta-Analysis. *Food Sci Nutr*. 2025 Dec 15;13(12):e71358.
[260] Sebo ZL, Rodeheffer MS. Testosterone metabolites differentially regulate obesogenesis and fat distribution. *Mol Metab*. 2020 Dec 9;44:101141.
[261] Mansoori A, Hosseini SA, Zilaee, et al. Effect of fenugreek extract supplement on testosterone levels in male: A meta-analysis of clinical trials. *Phytother Res*. 2020 Feb;34(7):1550-55.
[262] Kiss R, Szabo K, Gesztelyi R, et al. Insulin-Sensitizer Effects of Fenugreek Seeds in Parallel with Changes in Plasma MCH Levels in Healthy Volunteers. *Int J Mol Sci*. 2018;19(3):771.

[263] Talbott SM, Talbott JA, George A, et al. Effect of Tongkat Ali on stress hormones and psychological mood state in moderately stressed subjects. *J Int Soc Sports Nutr*. 2013;10(1):28.
[264] Chandrasekhar K, Kapoor J, Anishetty S. A prospective, randomized double-blind, placebo-controlled study of safety and efficacy of a high-concentration full-spectrum extract of ashwagandha root in reducing stress and anxiety in adults. *Indian J Psychol Med*. 2012;34(3):255-262.
[265] Smith SJ, Lopresti A, Teo SYM, et al. Examining the Effects of Herbs on Testosterone Concentrations in Men: A Systematic Review. *Adv Nutr*. 2021 May;12(3):744-65.
[266] Keller JL, Housh TJ, Hill EC, et al. The effects of Shilajit supplementation on fatigue-induced decreases in muscular strength and serum hydroxyproline levels. *J Int Soc Sports Nutr*. 2019 Feb 6;16:3.
[267] Pandit SL, Yaligar D, Halemane M, et al. A proprietary blend of standardized Punica granatum fruit rind and Theobroma cocoa seed extracts mitigates aging males' symptoms: A randomized, double-blind, placebo-controlled study. *Int J Med Sci*. 2022;19(8):1290-1299.
[268] Dalessandri KM, Firestone GL, Fitch MD, Bradlow HL, Bjeldanes LF. Pilot study: effect of 3,3'-diindolylmethane supplements on urinary hormone metabolites in postmenopausal women with a history of early-stage breast cancer. *Nutr Cancer*. 2004;50(2):161-167.
[269] van Die MD, Burger HG, Teede HJ, Bone KM. *Vitex agnus-castus* (Chaste-tree/berry) in the treatment of female reproductive disorders: a systematic review of randomized controlled trials. *Planta Med*. 2013;79(7):562-575.
[270] Steels E, Steele M, Harold M, et al. Efficacy of a Proprietary Trigonella foenum-graecum L. De-Husked Seed Extract in Reducing Menopausal Symptoms in Otherwise Healthy Women: A Double-Blind, Randomized, Placebo-Controlled Study. *Phytother Res*. 2017 sep;31(9):1316-22.
[271] Khanna A, Thomas J, John F, et al. Safety and influence of a novel extract of fenugreek on healthy young women: a randomized, double-blinded, placebo-controlled study. *Clin Phytosci*. 2021;7(63).
[272] Gopal S, Ajgaonkar A, Kanchi P, et al. Effect of an ashwagandha root extract (*Withania somnifera*) on sex hormones and perimenopausal symptoms: A randomized, double-blind, placebo-controlled study. *J Obstet Gynaecol Res*. 2021;47(12):4414-4423.
[273] Heger M, Ventskovskiy BM, Amar G, et al. Efficacy and tolerance of a special extract of *Rheum rhaponticum* in perimenopausal women with menopausal symptoms: a double-blind, placebo-controlled, 12-week project. *Maturitas*. 2006;55(3):235-244.
[274] Hasper I, Ventskovskiy BM, Rettenberger R, Heger PW, Kaszkin-Bettag M. Long-term efficacy and safety of the special extract ERr 731 of *Rheum rhaponticum* in perimenopausal women with menopausal symptoms. *Menopause*. 2009;16(1):117-131.

[275] Vollmer G, Papke A, Zierau O. Treatment of menopausal symptoms by an extract from the roots of rhapontic rhubarb: the role of estrogen receptors. *Chin Med.* 2010;5(1):7.
[276] Hajirahimkhan A, Dietz BM, Bolton JL. Botanical modulation of menopausal symptoms: mechanisms of action? *Planta Med.* 2013;79(7):538-553.
[277] Wober J, Möller F, Richter T, et al. Activation of estrogen receptor-beta by a special extract of *Rheum rhaponticum* (ERr 731), its aglycones and whole-body extracts from *Vitis vinifera. J Steroid Biochem Mol Biol.* 2007;107(3-5):191-201.
[278] Meissner HO, Mscisz A, Reich-Bilinska H, et al. Hormone-balancing effect of pre-gelatinized organic maca (*Lepidium meyenii*) in postmenopausal women. *Int J Biomed Sci.* 2006;2(4):375-394.
[279] Wichman J, Winther KH, Bonnema SJ, et al. Selenium supplementation significantly reduces thyroid antibody levels in patients with Hashimoto's thyroiditis: a systematic review and meta-analysis. *Thyroid.* 2016;26(12):1681-1692.
[280] Johnson SA. Medicinal Essential Oils: The Science and Practice of Evidence-Based Essential Oil Therapy (second edition). Scott A. Johnson Professional Writing Services, LLC; 2023.
[281] Johnson SA. Medicinal Essential Oils: The Science and Practice of Evidence-Based Essential Oil Therapy (second edition). Scott A. Johnson Professional Writing Services, LLC; 2023.
[282] Gertsch J, Leonti M, Raduner S, et al. Beta-caryophyllene is a dietary cannabinoid. *Proc Natl Acad Sci U S A.* 2008;105(26):11090-11095.
[283] Johnson SA. Beating Oxidative Stress Naturally. Scott A. Johnson Professional Writing Services, LLC; 2026.
[284] Johnson SA. Medicinal Essential Oils: The Science and Practice of Evidence-Based Essential Oil Therapy (second edition). Scott A. Johnson Professional Writing Services, LLC; 2023.
[285] Johnson SA. Medicinal Essential Oils: The Science and Practice of Evidence-Based Essential Oil Therapy (second edition). Scott A. Johnson Professional Writing Services, LLC; 2023.
[286] Handu D, Stote K, Piemonte T. Evaluating Bioactive-Substance-Based Interventions for Adults with MASLD: Results from a Systematic Scoping Review. *Nutrients.* 2025 Jan 26;17(3):453.
[287] Panyod S, Wu WK, Shieh YC, et al. Ginger essential oil prevents NASH progression by blocking the NLRP3 inflammasome and remodeling the gut microbiota-LPS-TLR4 pathway in mice. *Nutr Diabet.* 2024 Aug;14(65).
[288] Lai YS, Chen WC, Ho CT, et al. Garlic Essential Oil Protects against Obesity-Triggered Nonalcoholic Fatty Liver Disease through Modulation of Lipid Metabolism and Oxidative Stress. *J Agric Food Chem.* 2014 May;62(25):5897-5906.

[289] Johnson SA. Co2 Aromatics, Medicinal Herbs, and Targeted Nutraceuticals for Healing and Greater Wellness. Scott A. Johnson Professional Writing Services, LLC; 2023.
[290] Gong X, Su X, Liu H. Diallyl Trisulfide, the Antifungal Component of Garlic Essential Oil and the Bioactivity of Its Nanoemulsions Formed by Spontaneous Emulsification. *Molecules*. 2021 Nov;26(23):7186.
[291] BenchChem. Comparative Analysis of the Biological Activity of Diethyl Disulfide and Other Organosulfur
Compounds. 2026 Apr. CAS No.: 110-81-6.
[292] Lin H., Li Z, Sun Y, et al. D-Limonene: Promising and Sustainable Natural Bioactive Compound. *Appl Sci*. 2024;14(11):4605.
[293] Luo G, Fang F, Guo Y, et al. D-limonene modulates AMPK signaling to inhibit ox-LDL-induced foam cell formation. *Sci Rep*. 2026;16(22).
[294] Fan G, Wang Q, Li M, et al. Protective effect of orange essential oil in the formation of non-alcoholic fatty liver caused by high-fat diet. *Food Funct*. 2022 Jan;13(2).
[295] Asadollahpoor A, Abdollahi M, Rahimi R, et al. Pimpinella anisum L. fruit: Chemical composition and effect on rat model of nonalcoholic fatty liver disease. *J Res Med Sci*. 2017 Mar 15;22:37.
[296] Debnath I, Ghosh S, Bhunia S, et al. Mechanistic and clinical insights into the antidiabetic potential of Cinnamomum cassia: A review. *Pharmacol Res Nat Prod*. 2025 Sep;8:100340.
[297] Ping H, Zhang G, Ren G. Antidiabetic effects of cinnamon oil in diabetic KK-Ay mice. *Food Chem Toxicol*. 2010 Aug-Sep;48(8-9):2344-9.
[298] Johnson SA. Medicinal Essential Oils: The Science and Practice of Evidence-Based Essential Oil Therapy (second edition). Scott A. Johnson Professional Writing Services, LLC; 2023.
[299] Jafari S, Sattari R, Ghavamzadeh S, et al. Evaluation the effect of 50 and 100 mg doses of Cuminum cyminum essential oil on glycemic indices, insulin resistance and serum inflammatory factors on patients with diabetes type II: A double-blind randomized placebo-controlled clinical trial. *J Tradit Complement Med*. 2016 Dec 21;7(3):332-338.
[300] Morovati A, Pourghassem Gargari B, Sarbakhsh P, et al. The effect of cumin supplementation on metabolic profiles in patients with metabolic syndrome: A randomized, triple blind, placebocontrolled
clinical trial. *Phytother Res*. 2019 Apr;33(4):1182-1190.
[301] Johnson SA. Co2 Aromatics, Medicinal Herbs, and Targeted Nutraceuticals for Healing and Greater Wellness. Scott A. Johnson Professional Writing Services, LLC; 2023.
[302] Johnson SA. Medicinal Essential Oils: The Science and Practice of Evidence-Based Essential Oil Therapy (second edition). Scott A. Johnson Professional Writing Services, LLC; 2023.

[303] Diab F, Zbeeeb H, Zeaiter L, et al. Unraveling the metabolic activities of bioactive compounds on cellular models of hepatosteatosis and adipogenesis through docking analysis with PPARs. *Sci Rep*. 2024;14(28196).
[304] Donelli D, Antonelli M, Bellinazzi C, Gensini GF, Firenzuoli F. Effects of lavender on anxiety: A systematic review and meta-analysis. *Phytomedicine*. 2019;65:153099.
[305] Dold M, Bartova L, Volz HP, et al. Efficacy of Silexan in patients with anxiety disorders: a meta-analysis of randomized, placebo-controlled trials. *Eur Arch Psych Clin Neurosci*. 2023;273:1615-28.
[306] Milanos S, Elsharif S, Janzen D, et al. Metabolic Products of Linalool and Modulation of GABAA Receptors. *Front Chem*. 2017 Jun 21;5:46.
[307] Watanabe E, Kuchta K, Kimura M, et al. Effects of bergamot (Citrus bergamia Risso et Poiteau) essential oil aromatherapy on mood states, parasympathetic nervous system activity and salivary cortisol levels in 41 healthy females. *Forsch Komplementmed*. 2015;22(1):43-49.
[308] Moussaieff A, Rimmerman N, Bregman T, et al. Incensole acetate, an incense component, elicits psychoactivity by activating TRPV3 channels in the brain. *FASEB J*. 2008 Aug;22(8):3024–3034.
[309] Khanna R, MacDonald JK, Levesque BG. Peppermint oil for the treatment of irritable bowel syndrome: A systematic review and meta-analysis. *J Clin Gastroenterol*. 2014;48(6):505-512.
[310] El Jurdi K, Al Souky N, Melquist SJ. Efficacy of Peppermint Oil in Irritable Bowel Syndrome: A Systematic Review and Meta-Analysis. *Am J Gastroenterol*. 2023 Oct;118(10S):S498-9.
[311] Santiago MC, et al. Limonene activates PPAR-alpha and ameliorates hepatic steatosis in high-fat diet-induced obese mice. *Nutr Diabetes*. 2017;7(4):e262.
[312] Rambod M, Rakhshan M, Tohidinik S, et al. The effect of lemon inhalation aromatherapy on blood pressure, electrocardiogram changes, and anxiety in acute myocardial infarction patients: A clinical, multi-centered, assessor-blinded trial design. *Complement Ther Clin Pract*. 2020 May;39:101155.
[313] Goncalves S, Castro J, Almeida A, et al. A systematic review of the therapeutic properties of lemon essential oil. *Adv Integrative Med*. 2025 Sep;12(3):100433.
[314] Johnson SA. Co2 Aromatics, Medicinal Herbs, and Targeted Nutraceuticals for Healing and Greater Wellness. Scott A. Johnson Professional Writing Services, LLC; 2023.
[315] Newsome PN, Buchholtz K, Cusi K, et al. A placebo-controlled trial of subcutaneous semaglutide in nonalcoholic steatohepatitis. *N Engl J Med*. 2021;384(12):1113-1124.
[316] Long JD, Harrison SA, Newsome PN, et al. Semaglutide in the treatment of metabolic dysfunction-associated steatohepatitis: Results from the phase 3 ESSENCE trial. *N Engl J Med*. 2024;391(14):1210-1222.

[317] Hu Z, Tian D, Yang Z, et al. The mechanisms of GLP-1 receptor agonists in liver diseases: their multifaceted impact on immune response and metabolic regulation. *Front Pharmacol.* 2026 Mar;17:2026.
[318] Liao C, Liang X, Zhang X, et al. The effects of GLP-1 receptor agonists on visceral fat and liver ectopic fat in an adult population with or without diabetes and nonalcoholic fatty liver disease: A systematic review and meta-analysis. *PLoS One.* 2023 Aug 24;18(8):e0289616.
[319] Kazeminasab F, Kerchi AB, Sharafifard F, et al. The Effects of Creatine Supplementation on Upper- and Lower-Body Strength and Power: A Systematic Review and Meta-Analysis. *Nutrients.* 2025;17(17):2748.
[320] Bear DE, Langan A, Abu-Kummer E, et al. beta-Hydroxy-beta-methylbutyrate and its impact on skeletal muscle mass and function in clinical practice: a systematic review. *PLoS One.* 2019;14(6):e0212963. doi:10.1371/journal.pone.0212963
[321] Evans W, Shankaran M, Nyangau E, et al. Effects of Fortetropin on the Rate of Muscle Protein Synthesis in Older Men and Women: A Randomized, Double-Blinded, Placebo-Controlled Study. *J Gerontol A Biol Sci Med Sci.* 2021 Jan 1;76(1):108-114.
[322] MYOS MD. About Fortetropin. Accessed May 12, 2026 from: https://myosmd.com/pages/about-fortetropin.
[323] MYOS MD. Accessed May 12, 2026 from: https://myosmd.com/blogs/news/press-release-preserve-muscle-glp-1.
[324] Cusi K, Orsak B, Bril F, et al. Long-term pioglitazone treatment for patients with nonalcoholic steatohepatitis and prediabetes or type 2 diabetes: a randomized trial. *Ann Intern Med.* 2016;165(5):305-315.
[325] Belfort R, Harrison SA, Brown K, et al. A placebo-controlled trial of pioglitazone in subjects with nonalcoholic steatohepatitis. *N Engl J Med.* 2006;355(22):2297-2307.
[326] Musso G, Cassader M, Paschetta E, et al. Thiazolidinediones and PPIs in the treatment of nonalcoholic steatohepatitis: A meta-analysis of randomized controlled trials. *JAMA Internal Medicine.* 2011;171(16):1431-1440.
[327] Harrison SA, Bedossa P, Guyader D, et al. A phase 3, randomized, controlled trial of resmetirom in NASH with liver fibrosis. *N Engl J Med.* 2024;390(6):497-509.
[328] Zinman B, Wanner C, Lachin JM, et al. Empagliflozin, cardiovascular outcomes, and mortality in type 2 diabetes. *N Engl J Med.* 2015;373(22):2117-2128.
[329] Kumar N, Kumar B, Ashique S, et al. A critical review on SGLT2 inhibitors for diabetes mellitus, renal health, and cardiovascular conditions. *Diabetes Res Clin Pract.* 2025 Mar;221 (March 2025):112050.
[330] Abbas MS, Dandamudi M, Rehman T, et al. "Efficacy of SGLT2 inhibitors in non-diabetic non-alcoholic fatty liver disease: a systematic review and meta-analysis." *J Diabetes Metab Disord.* 2025 Dec 4;24(2):285.

[331] Haukeland JW, Konopski Z, Linnestad P, et al. Abnormal glucose tolerance is a predictor of nonalcoholic steatohepatitis and fibrosis in patients with nonalcoholic fatty liver disease. *Scand J Gastroenterol.* 2009;44(10):1192-1201.
[332] Musso G, Gambino R, Cassader M, et al. Meta-analysis: natural history of non-alcoholic fatty liver disease (NAFLD) and diagnostic accuracy of non-invasive tests for liver disease severity. *Ann Med.* 2011 Dec;43(8):617-49.
[333] Commins I, Clayton-Chubb D, Janko N, et al. Efficacy and Safety of Statins in MASLD and Other Chronic Liver Diseases. *Med Sci (Basel).* 2026 Feb 11;14(1):84.
[334] Sanyal AJ, Chalasani N, Kowdley KV, et al. Pioglitazone, vitamin E, or placebo for nonalcoholic steatohepatitis. *N Engl J Med.* 2010;362(18):1675-1685.
[335] Younossi ZM, Ratziu V, Loomba R, et al. Obeticholic acid for the treatment of non-alcoholic steatohepatitis: interim analysis from a multicentre, randomised, placebo-controlled, phase 3 trial. *The Lancet.* 2019;394(10215):2184-2196.
[336] Loomba R, Hartman ML, Aronne LJ, et al. Tirzepatide for the treatment of nonalcoholic steatohepatitis: A multicenter, randomized, double-blind, parallel-group, phase 2 trial (SYNERGY-NASH). *The Lancet.* 2024;403(10444):2601-2612.
[337] Wolfe MM, Boylan MO, Chin WW. Glucose-Dependent Insulinotropic Polypeptide in Incretin Physiology. *Endocrine Rev.* 2025 Feb;2025:bnaf006.
[338] Zhang Q, Delessa CT, Augustin R, et al. The glucose-dependent insulinotropic polypeptide (GIP) regulates body weight and food intake via CNS-GIPR signaling. *Cell Metab.* 2021 Apr;33(I4):833-44.
[339] Jastreboff AM, Aronne LJ, Ahmad NN, et al. Tirzepatide once weekly for the treatment of obesity. *N Engl J Med.* 2022;387(3):205-220.
[340] Ramos RAH, Hong I, Ortiz M, et al. Effects of Tirzepatide on Skeletal Muscle Mass in Adults: A Systematic Review. *Cureus.* 2025 Jul 29;17(7):e89020.
[341] Jastreboff AM, Kaplan LM, Frías JP, et al. Triple-hormone-receptor agonist retatrutide for obesity—a phase 2 trial. *N Engl J Med.* 2023;389(6):514-526.
[342] Jastreboff AM, Kaplan LM, Frías JP, et al; TRIUMPH-4 Investigators. Retatrutide for the treatment of obesity: 68-week results of a phase 3 randomized trial. *Lancet.* 2025;406(10512):1120-1134.
[343] Sanyal AJ, Frias JP, Hartman ML, et al. Triple hormone receptor agonist retatrutide for metabolic dysfunction-associated steatotic liver disease: a randomized phase 2a trial. *Nat Med.* 2024;30(6):1623-1633.
[344] Gao Y, Wei X, Wei P, et al. MOTS-c Functionally Prevents Metabolic Disorders. *Metabolites.* 2023 Jan 13;13(1):125.

345 Lee C, Zeng J, Drew BG, et al. The Mitochondrial-Derived Peptide MOTS-c Promotes Metabolic Homeostasis and Reduces Obesity and Insulin Resistance. *Cell Metab*. 2015 Mar;21(3):p443-54.
346 Thoudam T, Zeng G, Gao H, et al. Mitochondria-derived peptides in liver disease: Emerging regulators of hepatic metabolism and therapeutic targets. *Hepatol Commun*. 2026 Jan 9;10(2):e0885.
347 Zheng Y, Wei Z, Wang T. MOTS-c: A promising mitochondrial-derived peptide for therapeutic exploitation. *Front Endocrinol (Lausanne)*. 2023 Jan 25;14:1120533.
348 Alzheimer's Drug Discovery Foundation. MOTS-c. 2025 Sep 17.
349 Harrison SA, et al. Efruxifermin in non-alcoholic steatohepatitis with F2 or F3 fibrosis (HARMONY): a multicentre, randomised, double-blind, placebo-controlled, phase 2b trial. *Lancet Gastroenterol Hepatol*. 2023.
350 Loomba R, et al. Randomized, controlled trial of the FGF21 analogue pegozafermin in NASH. *N Engl J Med*. 2023;389:998-1011.
351 Chang E, Zhu Y, Wei W, et al. Chiglitazar, a PPAR pan-agonist: Impacts on type 2 diabetes mellitus and multi-system metabolic regulation–A review. *Biomed Pharmacother*. 2025 Dec;193:118850.
352 Mandal SK, Muzaffar-Ur-Rehman M, Puri S, et al. In silico and in vitro investigations reveal pan-PPAR agonist activity and anti-NAFLD efficacy of polydatin by modulating hepatic lipid-energy metabolism. *Sci Rep*. 2025 Jul;15(26995).
353 Cooreman MP, Butler J, Giugliano RP, et al. The pan-PPAR agonist lanifibranor improves cardiometabolic health in patients with metabolic dysfunction-associated steatohepatitis. *Natur Commun*. 2024 May;15(3962).
354 Zeevi D, Korem T, Zmora N, et al. Personalized nutrition by prediction of glycemic responses. *Cell*. 2015;163(5):1079-1094.
355 Saliba-Gustafsson P, Hardfeldt J, Pederelli M, et al. Genomic Signatures of MASLD: How Genomics Is Redefining Our Understanding of Metabolic Liver Disease. *Int J Mol Sci*. 2025;26(22):10881.
356 Liao X, Li Y, Tang S, et al. Continuous glucose monitoring in non-diabetic populations: a systematic review of observational and interventional studies with meta-analysis. *Eur J Med Res*. 2026;31(397).
357 Huh KY, Oh J, Lee S, et al. Clinical Evaluation of Digital Therapeutics: Present and Future. *Healthc Inform Res*. 2022 Jul 31;28(3):188–197.
358 Xu X, Jiang L, Wu C, et al. The role of fibrosis index FIB-4 in predicting liver fibrosis stage and clinical prognosis: A diagnostic or screening tool? *J Formosan Med Assoc*. 2022 Feb;121(2):454-66.

Index

F

G

H

I

K

L

M

N

O

P

R

S

T

U

V

W

Appendices

www.ingramcontent.com/pod-product-compliance
Lightning Source LLC
LaVergne TN
LVHW010712061126
851857LV00014B/1143